Pan-cancer Integrative Molecular Portrait Towards a New Paradigm in Precision Medicine

Christophe Le Tourneau • Maud Kamal

Editors

Pan-cancer Integrative Molecular Portrait Towards a New Paradigm in Precision Medicine

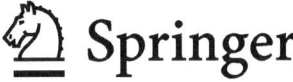 Springer

Editors

Christophe Le Tourneau
Institut Curie
Department of Medical Oncology
Saint-Cloud, Paris
France

Maud Kamal
Institut Curie
Department of Medical Oncology
Saint-Cloud, Paris
France

ISBN 978-3-319-22188-5   ISBN 978-3-319-22189-2   (eBook)
DOI 10.1007/978-3-319-22189-2

Library of Congress Control Number: 2015949934

Springer Cham Heidelberg New York Dordrecht London

Printed on acid-free paper

Springer International Publishing AG Switzerland is part of Springer Science+Business Media
(www.springer.com)

Contents

Contributors

Bernard Asselain, MD, PhD Biostatistics Department, INSERM U900, Institut Curie, Paris, France

Ivan Bièche, PharmD, PhD Department of Genetics, Institut Curie, Paris, France

EA7331, University of Paris-Descartes, Paris, France

Céline Callens, PharmD, PhD Department of Genetics, Institut Curie, Paris, France

Thomas Rio Frio, PhD Genoma SA, NGS Platform, Geneva, Switzerland

David Gentien Translational Research Department, Institut Curie, Paris, France

Philippe Hupé, PhD Bioinformatics Platform, Institut Curie, Paris, France

Unité INSERM/Institut Curie U900, Paris, France

Maud Kamal, PhD Department of Medical Oncology, Institut Curie, Saint-Cloud, Paris, France

Xavier Paoletti, PhD Biostatistics and Epidemiology Department, INSERM U1018, Villejuif, France

Gaëlle Pierron, PhD Department of Genetics, Institut Curie, Paris, France

Cécile Reyes Translational Research Department, Institut Curie, Paris, France

Etienne Rouleau, PharmD, PhD Department of Genetics, Institut Curie, Paris, France

Nicolas Servant Bioinformatics Platform, Institut Curie, Paris, France

Unité INSERM/Institut Curie U900, Paris, France

Christophe Le Tourneau, MD, PhD Department of Medical Oncology, Institut Curie, Saint-Cloud, Paris, France

EA7285, Versailles-Saint-Quentin-en-Yvelines University, Versailles, France

Anne Vincent-Salomon, MD, PhD Department of Pathology, Institut Curie, Paris, France

Abbreviations

APS	Adenosine 5′-phosphosulfate
AR	Androgen receptor
BAC	Bacterial artificial chromosome
BRCs	Biological resources centers
BWT	Burrows-Wheeler transform
CDS	Clinical decision support
CGH	Comparative genomic hybridization
CNVs	Copy number variations
COSMIC	The Catalogue of Somatic Mutations in Cancer
ctDNA	Circulating tumoral DNA
ddNTP	Dideoxynucleotide triphosphate
dNTP	Deoxynucleotide triphosphate
EHR	Electronic health record
ER	Estrogen receptors
EVS	Exome Variant Server
FFPE	Formalin-fixed paraffin-embedded
FISH	Fluorescent in situ hybridization
FITC	Fluorescein isothiocyanate
GATK	Genome Analysis Toolkit
gDNA	Genomic DNA
GoF	Gain of function
Her2	Human epidermal growth factor receptor 2 (ERBB2)
HGP	Human Genome project
HGVS	Human Genome Variation Society
ICGC	International Cancer Genome Consortium
IHC	Immunohistochemistry
Indel	Insertions or deletions
LINE	Long interspersed nuclear elements
LoF	Loss of function
MAF	Minor allele frequency
MAQ	Mapping quality score

MBB	Molecular biology board
MeDIP-seq	Methylated-DNa immunoprecipitation
MIP	Molecular inversion probes
MTA	Molecularly targeted agents
NGS	Next-generation sequencing
NIPT	Noninvasive prenatal testing
OS	Overall survival
PAC	Plasmid artificial chromosome
PCR	Polymerase chain reaction
PFS	Progression-free survival
PM	Precision medicine
PR	Progesterone receptor
RMH	Royal Marsden Hospital
SINE	Short interspersed nuclear elements
SNP	Single nucleotide polymorphisms
SNV	Single nucleotide variant
SOLiD	Sequencing by oligonucleotide ligation and detection
SVs	Structural variants
TCGA	The Cancer Genome Atlas
TdT	Terminal deoxynucleotidyl transferase
TME	Tumor microenvironment
TSG	Tumor suppressor gene
TTP	Time to progression
UNC	University of North Carolina
VCF	Variant calling format
WES	Whole exome sequencing
WGA	Whole genome amplification
YAC	Yeast artificial chromosome

Chapter 1
Introduction: Rationale for Precision Medicine Clinical Trials

Christophe Le Tourneau

1.1 Introduction

A normal cell becomes a cancer cell following successive genomic alterations. Cancer is therefore considered as a genomic disease. The identification of genomic alterations in the tumor genome leading to tumor proliferation has led to the development of molecularly targeted agents (MTAs). MTAs block a peculiar molecular alteration involved in cell proliferation, angiogenesis, metastasis, invasion, etc. The development of some of these agents in molecularly defined subgroups of patients has yielded unprecedented efficacy in some tumor types (Shaw et al. 2013; Sosman et al. 2012; Druker et al. 2001; Sekulic et al. 2012; Slamon et al. 2011; Maemondo et al. 2010). The concept of personalized medicine has arisen in oncology with the emergence of MTAs 15 years ago. Personalized medicine, also called precision medicine, is defined by the National Cancer Institute as "A form of medicine that uses information about a person's genes, proteins, and environment to prevent, diagnose, and treat disease."

Although some molecular alterations have been reported across different tumor types, MTAs have followed the same clinical development as cytotoxic agents based on tumor location and histology (Fig. 1.1) (Ciriello et al. 2013). A retrospective review of refractory cancer patients included in phase I trials at the MD Anderson Cancer Center reported that the response to treatment was higher in patients treated with an MTA that matched a molecular alteration identified in the tumor, independent of tumor location and histology (Tsimberidou et al. 2012). The emergence of

C. Le Tourneau, MD, PhD
Department of Medical Oncology, Institut Curie, Saint-Cloud, Paris, France

EA7285, Versailles-Saint-Quentin-en-Yvelines University, Versailles, France
e-mail: christophe.letourneau@curie.fr

© Springer International Publishing Switzerland 2015
C. Le Tourneau, M. Kamal (eds.), *Pan-cancer Integrative Molecular Portrait Towards a New Paradigm in Precision Medicine*,
DOI 10.1007/978-3-319-22189-2_1

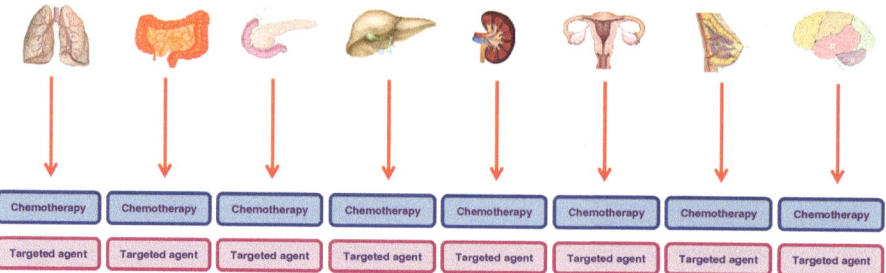

Fig. 1.1 Current way of developing anticancer drugs

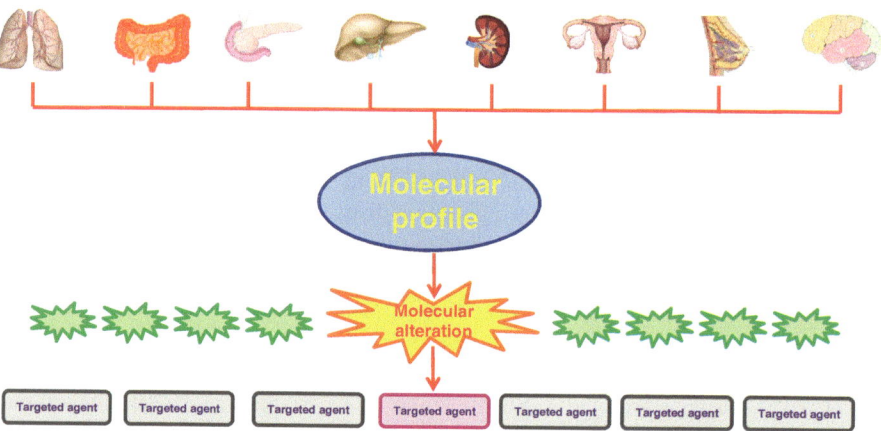

Fig. 1.2 Concept of precision medicine

MTAs has not immediately led to a paradigm shift in drug development for the following reasons: (1) Molecular alterations were initially thought to be specific of certain tumor types, such as the *BCR/ABL* fusion gene in chronic myeloid leukemia; (2) the functional significance of some molecular alterations varies across tumor types, as illustrated by the limited efficacy of *BRAF* inhibitors in *BRAF* V600E-mutated colorectal cancer (Prahallad et al. 2012) and the substantial efficacy of these drugs in *BRAF* V600E-mutated melanoma (Sosman et al. 2012); (3) histology-independent drug development would be challenged by the lack of valid benchmarks represented by data on drug efficacy in patients with any type of cancer harboring a common molecular alteration.

Since recently, advances in high-throughput technologies have allowed depicting most druggable molecular alterations for an affordable cost in a time frame compatible with clinical practice. Despite the caveats associated with histology-independent drug development mentioned above, the question whether precision medicine based on the molecular profiling of the tumor of cancer patients would still improve their outcome has arisen and led to set up clinical trials addressing this question (Fig. 1.2). These clinical trials evaluate a treatment algorithm instead of drug efficacy. These studies are associated with numerous challenges that are later discussed.

1.2   Personalized Medicine Trials

One fundamental requirement in these precision medicine trials is that the treatment algorithm is not modified during the study. These trials include nonrandomized trials that usually use patients as their own control to assess efficacy, and randomized trials that address various questions. All these trials have been set up in the metastatic setting, either in patients with refractory cancers or as maintenance therapy. If the precision medicine concept is validated, it will have to be evaluated at earlier stages of the disease.

Von Hoff's study was the first published histology-independent clinical trial using tumor molecular alterations to select treatment (von Hoff et al. 2010). Patients with any type of recurrent and/or metastatic cancer that was refractory to standard of care had selected molecular alterations analyzed using immunohistochemistry (IHC), FISH, and oligonucleotide microarray gene expression assays. Based on the detected molecular alterations, a drug or drug combination was prescribed. Efficacy was assessed using each patient as his own control by determining the time of disease control on the treatment guided by the molecular profile compared to the time of disease control on the last treatment. Disease control was assessed using well-established criteria to measure progression-free survival (PFS). Eighteen of the 66 treated patients (27 %) had a ratio of the PFS on matching targeted treatment to the PFS under the last previous treatment >1.3, which was considered a positive result. More recently, the WIN Consortium launched the WINTHER trial (NCT01856296) which is similar to von Hoff's study in its concept (http://www.cancer.gov/clinical-trials/search/view?cdrid=749710&version=HealthProfessional&protocolsearc hid=12176033). This trial is open to patients with any kind of refractory advanced cancer. Two samples are taken from the patient, the first one from a metastatic site and the second from adjacent normal tissue. Druggable molecular alterations are first investigated from the tumor sample using next-generation sequencing (NGS) for mutations screening and comparative genomic hybridization (CGH) array for gene copy number variations. If a druggable molecular alteration is identified, patients are either guided to a phase I clinical trial with an agent presumably matching the molecular alteration or are being prescribed an already approved MTA off-label. If no druggable molecular alteration is detected, data from tumoral RNA and RNA from normal adjacent tissue are analyzed in order to identify gene expression profiles that can orient the patient to the best therapy. Both treatment arms will be analyzed separately using PFS ratio as a primary end point. The main advantage of this trial is that all included patients will be treated. Given the multiple tumor types included in these nonrandomized trials, one way to evaluate treatment efficacy has been to use patients as their own controls assessing the PFS ratio. The main criticism to the use of the PFS ratio as a primary end point in these studies is the assessment of PFS on the last therapy outside of the clinical trial. In addition, the underlying assumption behind this end point is that the natural history of disease is linear over time, in other words that the two PFS are correlated, which might not be true. For these reasons, the use of randomization has been suggested (Doroshow 2010).

The SHIVA trial (NCT01771458) was a proof-of-concept randomized phase II trial comparing molecularly targeted therapy based on tumor molecular profiling *versus* conventional chemotherapy in patients with any type of cancer that was refractory to standard of care (Le Tourneau et al. 2012a). The primary end point was PFS. Given the heterogeneity in terms of prognosis of patients with various tumor types, the trial was stratified on (1) the patient's prognosis using the Royal Marsden Hospital prognostic score for refractory cancer patients (Arkenau et al. 2009) and (2) the signaling pathway, the selected molecular alteration belongs to. Molecular alterations were evaluated on a tumor sample from a metastatic site using NGS for mutations screening, CytoScan HD for gene copy number variations, and IHC for estrogen, progesterone, and androgen receptor expression analyses. Only marketed MTAs were used in this trial according to a prespecified treatment algorithm. Eleven MTAs were available within the clinical trial, whereas conventional chemotherapy was prescribed at the physician's discretion in the control arm. Crossover was proposed in both arms at disease progression, allowing the evaluation of tumor growth kinetics on both treatments for each patient (Le Tourneau et al. 2012b). Physicians were being told the molecular alteration of interest for their patient only at the time the patients were about to be treated in the experimental arm. Feasibility results on the first 100 included patients have shown that biopsies are safe and that at least one molecular alteration was detected in 40 % of patients allowing them to be randomized (Le Tourneau et al. 2014). Ancillary studies include the evaluation of the ability of circulating DNA to predict treatment efficacy or resistance, as well as a medico-economic evaluation of the experimental strategy. Efficacy results showed a differential effect depending on the signaling pathway (Le Tourneau et al. 2015). While the overall result was negative, patients treated with MTAs targeting the RAF/MEK pathway had a longer PFS in the experimental arm (3.7 months as compared to 2.0 months). This suggests that the precision medicine approach might be valid in this subgroup. This will be evaluated in the SHIVA02 trial that should start in 2016.

The MPACT trial is an ongoing randomized phase II trial led by the National Cancer Institute that includes as the same patient population the SHIVA trial (Kummar ASCO meeting 2013). A tumor sample of a metastatic site is also mandatory. Molecular alterations are detected using similar technologies as in the SHIVA trial. Patients are randomized between therapy matching the detected molecular alteration and therapy not matching the detected molecular alteration. Crossover is proposed at disease progression for patients randomized in the nonmatching treatment arm. Although it might be difficult for patients to accept the randomization in the nonmatching treatment arm, this design is the only one that evaluates solely the treatment algorithm. Accrual has started in 2014.

The MOST trial (EudraCT: 2012-004510-34) is a randomized discontinuation trial for patients who have progressed on first-line treatment for a recurrent and/or metastatic cancer led by the Centre Léon Bérard in Lyon (http://www.cancer-lyric.com/programme/programme-1/). Molecular alterations are identified on a sample from either a metastatic site or the primary tumor using similar technologies as in the previous trials. Patients are treated during 3 months with one of the five available already marketed MTAs. Responding patients will continue on therapy, while progressive patients will be taken off study. Patients with stable disease are randomized between treatment continuation and discontinuation for 2 months. The MOST trial will provide a more accurate evaluation of efficacy than a single-arm study by deciphering between disease stabilization related to the natural history of the disease and disease stabilization related to a cytostatic effect of molecularly targeted therapy. The trial has started in 2014.

The SAFIR 02 trials are tumor-specific randomized trials evaluating maintenance therapy (Andre et al. 2014). SAFIR 02 Breast includes patients with HER-2-negative and estrogen receptor-positive recurrent and/or metastatic breast cancer who have not progressed after four to eight cycles of first- or second-line chemotherapy, while SAFIR 02 Lung includes patients with *EGFR* and *ALK* wild-type recurrent and/or metastatic lung cancer who have not progressed after four cycles of first-line platinum-based chemotherapy. All patients have a tumor sample taken from a metastatic site in order to seek molecular alterations using the same technologies. Patients are randomized between an MTA from AstraZeneca matching the detected molecular alteration and maintenance chemotherapy. The primary end point is PFS. These trials have opened in 2014 as well. These trials evaluate the utility of a treatment algorithm for selecting maintenance therapy following first-line therapy in recurrent and/or metastatic luminal breast cancer and lung cancer not eligible for molecularly targeted therapy.

1.3 Perspectives

All these personalized medicine clinical trials base their algorithm on DNA analysis, except the WINTHER trial that also analyzes gene expression in case no molecular alteration is detected on DNA. These trials ultimately address with different angles the question of whether the use of tumor molecular profiling would improve patients' outcome. The SHIVA trial has opened the door to this approach with encouraging results. Results of the other trials are highly expected as they will provide meaningful information as to whether high-throughput technologies should or should not be used in routine in the future. None of these trials are powered to adequately assess the efficacy of any treatment in any molecularly defined subgroup of patients with a same tumor type and histology.

Given their complexity, precision medicine trials are associated with numerous challenges. These trials indeed involve several different crucial stakeholders, including physicians, radiologists, pathologists, biostatisticians, molecular screening platforms managers, bioinformaticians, and biologists. While the four former ones had been used to work together in a clinical setting, the latter ones usually worked with researchers and were not used to time constraints related to patient care. The novelty with precision medicine trials is that all these people have had to coordinate their actions so that treatment decisions for cancer patients are timely taken.

The emergence of cytotoxic chemotherapy after the Second World War has led to a significant improvement in cancer cure. While molecularly targeted therapy has clearly modified the prognostic of some cancers such as chronic myeloid leukemia or HER-2-overexpressing breast cancer, the cure rates of cancer patients have not substantially increased. Two reasons may explain this. First, a minority of cancer patients is today eligible for molecularly targeted therapy. Second, molecularly targeted therapy is mostly approved in the recurrent and/or metastatic setting where they prolong survival but do not cure. Only trastuzumab in HER-2-overexpressing breast cancer and imatinib in c-KIT-overexpressing gastrointestinal stromal tumors are approved in the adjuvant setting (Piccart-Gebhart et al. 2005; Dematteo et al. 2009). The substantial decrease of recurrences in these two settings likely provides an indirect demonstration that these two agents are able to cure cancer. The fundamental question we have today is whether the use of high-throughput technologies will increase the rate of cancer cure. The precision medicine trials described above are almost all performed in patients with recurrent and/or metastatic cancer and will certainly not lead to an increased cure rate of cancer. Only the evaluation of such strategies at earlier stages of the disease could potentially lead to substantially improve the rate of cancer cure. While positive results of these trials would undoubtedly accelerate the implementation of high-throughput screening technologies as routine, negative results should not be interpreted as a failure of the overall strategy. Subgroup analyses might also pinpoint potential biomarkers that might after clinical validation improve treatment efficacy when taken into account. Patients are indeed usually heavily pretreated in these trials. In addition, patients are usually proposed single-agent molecularly targeted therapy, which we know is often insufficient to achieve prolonged efficacy. Lastly, the treatment algorithms used in these trials have not been validated. Bioinformatics and research in biology will be critical to improve them, using systems biology approaches, along with functional validation in preclinical studies.

The precision medicine trials described above focus on the use of genomic alterations to decide molecularly targeted therapy. Other approaches to treat cancer have recently emerged and appear to be very promising, including immunotherapy and therapies targeting the microenvironment. Restoring an efficient immune response by targeting CTLA4 in melanoma patients has been demonstrated to improve their outcome in the recurrent and/or metastatic setting (Hodi et al. 2010). Up to 10 % of patients are long responders to this treatment, which is unprecedented. The future will tell whether they are cured, which might be plausible given the mechanism of action of these drugs. Outstanding results have also been reported in several tumor types with drugs targeting the PD-L1/*PD1* axis (Topalian et al. 2012; Brahmer et al. 2012; Hamid et al. 2013). Other drugs that target the microenvironment such anti-CSF-1R antibodies that target activated macrophages on the surface of which CSF-1R is present are in clinical development. Ultimately, it is very likely that the cure of cancer will substantially increase thanks to a combination of molecularly targeted therapy that will be more adequately used using high-throughput technologies and novel therapies such as immunotherapy and therapies targeting the microenvironment. The integration of these latter therapies to molecularly targeted therapy opens an important field in cancer research. The development of ctDNA will hopefully also help circumvent the issue of intratumor heterogeneity (Gerlinger et al. 2012).

References

Andre F, Bachelot T, Commo F et al (2014) Comparative genomic hybridisation array and DNA sequencing to direct treatment of metastatic breast cancer: a multicentre, prospective trial (SAFIR01/UNICANCER). Lancet Oncol 15:267–274

Arkenau HT, Barriuso J, Olmos D et al (2009) Prospective validation of a prognostic score to improve patient selection for oncology phase I trials. J Clin Oncol 27:2692–2696

Brahmer JR, Tykodi SS, Chow LQ et al (2012) Safety and activity of anti-PD-L1 antibody in patients with advanced cancer. N Engl J Med 366:2455–2465

Ciriello G, Miller ML, Aksoy BA, Senbabaoglu Y, Schultz N, Sander C (2013) Emerging landscape of oncogenic signatures across human cancers. Nat Genet 45:1127–1133

Dematteo RP, Ballman KV, Antonescu CR et al (2009) Adjuvant imatinib mesylate after resection of localised, primary gastrointestinal stromal tumor: a randomised, double-blind, placebo-controlled trial. Lancet 373:1097–1104

Doroshow JH (2010) Selecting systemic cancer therapy one patient at a time: is there a role for molecular profiling of individual patients with advanced solid tumors? J Clin Oncol 28:4869–4871

Druker BJ, Talpaz M, Resta DJ et al (2001) Efficacy and safety of a specific inhibitor of the BCR-ABL tyrosine kinase in chronic myeloid leukemia. N Engl J Med 344:1031–1037

Gerlinger M, Rowan AJ, Horswell S et al (2012) Intratumor heterogeneity and branched evolution revealed by multiregion sequencing. N Engl J Med 366:883–892

Hamid O, Robert C, Daud A et al (2013) Safety and tumor responses with lambrolizumab (anti-PD-1) in melanoma. N Engl J Med 369:134–144

Hodi FS, O'Day SJ, McDermott DF et al (2010) Improved survival with ipilimumab in patients with metastatic melanoma. N Engl J Med 363:711–723

Kummar S (2013) Molecular Profiling based Assignment of Cancer Therapy (MPACT). Proc NCI-EORT-ASCO meeting

Le Tourneau C, Kamal M, Trédan O et al (2012a) Designs and challenges for personalized medicine studies in oncology: focus on the SHIVA trial. Target Oncol 7:253–265

Le Tourneau C, Servois V, Diéras V et al (2012b) Tumor growth kinetics assessment: added value to RECIST in cancer patients treated with molecularly targeted agents. Br J Cancer 106:854–857

Le Tourneau C, Mitry E, Goncalves A et al (2014) Randomized phase II trial comparing therapy based on tumor molecular profiling versus conventional therapy in patients with refractory cancer: results of the feasibility part of the SHIVA trial. Br J Cancer 111:17–24

Le Tourneau C, Delord J.-P, Gonçalves A (2015) Randomized trial comparing molecularly targeted therapy based on tumor molecular profiling with conventional therapy in advanced cancer (SHIVA), Lancet Oncology, (in press)

Maemondo M, Inoue A, Kobayashi K et al (2010) Gefitinib or chemotherapy for non-small-cell lung cancer with mutated EGFR. N Engl J Med 362:2380–2388

Piccart-Gebhart MJ, Procter M, Leyland-Jones B et al (2005) Trastuzumab after adjuvant chemotherapy in HER2-positive breast cancer. N Engl J Med 353:1659–1672

Prahallad A, Sun C, Huang S et al (2012) Unresponsiveness of colon cancer to BRAF(V600E) inhibition through feedback activation of EGFR. Nature 483:100–103

Sekulic A, Migden MR, Oro AE et al (2012) Efficacy and safety of vismodegib in advanced basal-cell carcinoma. N Engl J Med 366:2171–2179

Shaw AT, Kim DW, Nakagawa K et al (2013) Crizotinib versus chemotherapy in advanced *ALK*-positive lung cancer. N Engl J Med 368:2385–2394

Slamon D, Eiermann W, Robert N et al (2011) Adjuvant trastuzumab in HER2-positive breast cancer. N Engl J Med 365:1273–2183

Sosman JA, Kim KB, Schuchter L et al (2012) Survival in *BRAF* V600-mutant advanced melanoma treated with vemurafenib. N Engl J Med 366:707–714

Topalian SL, Hodi FS, Brahmer JR et al (2012) Safety, activity, and immune correlates of anti-PD-1 antibody in cancer. N Engl J Med 366:2443–2454

Tsimberidou AM, Iskander NG, Hong DS et al (2012) Personalized medicine in a phase I clinical trials program: the MD Anderson Cancer Center Initiative. Clin Cancer Res 18:6373–6383

Von Hoff DD, Stephenson JJ, Rosen P et al (2010) Pilot study using molecular profiling of patients' tumors to find potential targets and select treatments for their refractory cancers. J Clin Oncol 28:4877–4883

Chapter 2
The Key Role of Pathology in the Context of Precision Medicine Trials

Anne Vincent-Salomon

2.1 Introduction

Pathology in the era of precision medicine highlights the complementarity between anatomic surgical pathology and genomics. Diagnosis in surgical pathology integrates the medical history of the patient's disease together with the anatomic modification of the ill organ and the microscopic tissue alteration. From a detailed and precise examination, the pathologist formulates diagnostic hypotheses that will be further confirmed with a combination of phenotypical patterns together with molecular alterations. Pathology is now considered a "crossover" discipline. It is multidisciplinary in nature and focuses mainly on the submicroscopic aspects of disease. A key consideration is that more accurate diagnosis is possible when the diagnosis is based on both the morphologic changes in tissues (traditional anatomic pathology) and on molecular testing. However, a molecular alteration can be shared by different tumor types such as *B-RAF* mutations that can be observed in cutaneous melanomas, colon cancers, and histiocytosis. Pathological analyses participate in getting insight into the molecular portrait of cancers and in adding information for the best therapeutic decisions.

Tissues submitted to pathological analyses in the context of precision medicine can be either the primary tumor or the metastatic disease. In both situations, pathologists adapt the level of information they can get from tissue examination. In between physicians and researchers, the pathologists are in the hub of translational research.

A. Vincent-Salomon, MD, PhD
Department of Pathology, Institut Curie, Paris, France
e-mail: anne.salomon@curie.fr

© Springer International Publishing Switzerland 2015
C. Le Tourneau, M. Kamal (eds.), *Pan-cancer Integrative Molecular Portrait Towards a New Paradigm in Precision Medicine*,
DOI 10.1007/978-3-319-22189-2_2

Below, we will briefly unravel the key steps of the pathological analyses useful for precision medicine.

2.2 Tissue Handling and Processing

2.2.1 Biopsy Sampling

Biopsies are by definition a sampling of the observed lesions. In order to confirm a metastatic disease progression, a biopsy of the lesions is sometimes performed. The radiologist works together with the pathologist to obtain the most representative samples of the lesions. To minimize the sampling issues, several biopsies of the same lesion are obtained whenever it's feasible. One of these samples is immediately snap-frozen in liquid nitrogen (-196 °C) and stored until nucleic acid extraction procedure. The other samples are quickly fixed in 10 % neutral-buffered formalin for pathological and subsequent molecular analyses.

2.2.2 Surgical Specimen

When it's clinically useful to consider a surgical treatment for the metastatic lesion, the pathologist has access to large amounts of tumor's tissues with the surgical specimen.

Preanalytical steps have to be standardized to enable all analyses including pathological analyses under the microscope to nucleic acid extractions. The key point is the shortest delay between surgical ischemia and fixation. The time to fixation has to be recorded. Before fixation, the surgical specimen is examined in details (weight, size) and pictures of this fresh surgical specimen are recorded. Frozen samples are taken in the most representative area of the tumor together with peri-tumoral normal tissue. Whenever possible, a fragment is fixed in formalin to keep a mirror formalin-fixed paraffin-embedded (FFPE) tumor block of the tumor area in which a frozen sample has been taken.

2.3 Sample Processing Before Molecular Analyses

2.3.1 Diagnosis

Surgical pathology analysis is performed in order to confirm the suspected diagnosis of disease. This is a mandatory step before any molecular analysis is performed. When the primary tumor has been diagnosed in the same laboratory, it is a good practice to compare the two lesions to appreciate similarities and differences that might be a consequence of intra-tumor heterogeneity.

2.3.2   Phenotyping

The comparison between the primary tumor and the metastasis helps to affiliate the two diseases. For example, hormonal receptors and HER2 expression are systematically analyzed on a suspected metastatic lesion of a breast carcinoma.

2.3.3   Cellularity Assessment

The tumor cellularity is performed on the FFPE and the frozen specimens. The most representative FFPE bloc of the metastasis is recorded in order to facilitate any further molecular analyses based on the nucleic acids extracted from this bloc.

The respective percentage of tumor cells; the percentage of in situ *versus* invasive lesions, of lymphoid infiltrates, and of (myo)-fibroblasts; and the existence of necrosis areas are taken into account.

2.3.4   Macrodissection for Tumor Cell Enrichment

Macrodissection is performed if necessary to enrich the tumor samples with tumoral cells before nucleic acid extraction. Macrodissection is a dissection performed without a microscope and refers to gross manual dissection of a frozen tissue sample embedded in OCT or a fixed tissue sample embedded in paraffin guided by a histologic section. A pathologist analyzes the histologic section in order to identify areas of the specimen containing the tumoral tissue and marks the guide slide accordingly. The marked guide slide is used by the technician to isolate those portions of the sample.

Three different methods of macrodissection exist: (1) block trimming method, (2) target tissue dissection method, and (3) tissue microarray needle-guided biopsy within a FFPE block. The choice of method depends on the characteristics of the particular target tissue and the particular tissue sample to ensure the greatest yield and enrichment of target cells and on experience of the technician who performs the macrodissection as well as the specific requirements of the nucleic acid extraction protocol. The block trimming method is best used when the target tissue makes up a fairly separated area and uniform proportion of the tissue specimen. It is also the method of choice for frozen specimens. The target tissue dissection method is best used when the target tissue makes up small discrete areas (only a few mm in diameter) in the tissue sample.

A pathologist examines a histologic section of the embedded tissue microscopically and circles, on the section with an indelible marker, the area(s) of target tissue that meets the requirement of the study. Using the circled histologic sections as a guide, the target areas are then dissected from the tissue using a pointed scalpel blade, generally incising into the tissue for a depth of approximately 2 mm. The dissected area is then collected into an appropriately sized sealable tube.

Though better defined than a non-dissected tissue sample, the actual percentage of targeted cells obtained by macrodissection can only be proscribed to the degree that tissue architecture and admixed cellular components allow. This will vary from tissue type to tissue type and from case to case. Although the percentage of target tissue can be estimated with a greater degree of precision than with a non-dissected tissue sample, this is still an estimate and not an absolute quantification of captured tissue.

2.4 In Situ Confirmation of Genomic Alterations

To confirm genomic alterations such as losses and amplifications that might have been identified during genomic analyses, immunohistochemistry (IHC) and in situ hybridization are powerful tools to validate the observed molecular alterations. These in situ techniques give a robust view of intra-tumoral heterogeneity. When antibodies specific of the protein of the altered gene exist, it facilitates the validation of a genomic loss of an amplification associated with the protein overexpression. A complete absence of expression of a protein within the tumoral cells is required to validate a genomic loss of its coding gene. Internal positive control is necessary to accurately interpret the staining. For example, the genomic loss or deletion of *PTEN* has been validated in the SHIVA trial using IHC (Le Tourneau et al. 2014) (Fig. 2.1). The monoclonal antibody specific of the *PTEN* amino acids 321–336 has been used (Zymed® laboratories). The internal control was a positive expression of *PTEN* in the stromal fibroblasts. A normal prostate tissue was used for an external control in every manipulation. Interpretation of the staining determined the percentage of tumoral positive cells, the intensity of the staining on a three-tiered scale (forms 1 to 3), as well as the good quality of the external control and the presence of the internal control.

Nuclear expression of *PTEN* has been reported but was not considered in the frame of the SHIVA trial for *PTEN* expression levels' interpretation. The cutoff to consider a case positive was at least 10 % of positive cells with a weak intensity. In the SHIVA trial, 7 cases presented a *PTEN* deletion and 100 a *PTEN* loss. One hundred three cases were available for *PTEN* IHC analysis. In 56 out of the 103 analyzed cases (54 %), *PTEN* was not expressed, signing out the genomic loss (Fig 2.2).

Genomic amplification or gains are associated with RNA and protein overexpression in 40 % of the cases. IHC or in situ hybridization is useful to gain insight into the biological significance of the genomic alteration. HER2 is the best example of amplification being associated in the vast majority of the cases with protein overexpression.

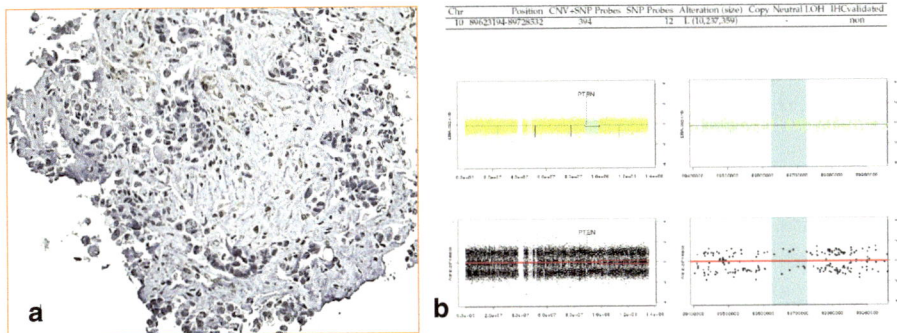

Fig. 2.1 Example of a *PTEN* loss of expression validating a *PTEN* genomic loss. (**a**) Immunolabeling of *PTEN* protein (clone A2B1, Zymed® laboratories, CA, USA). The metastatic cells are *PTEN* negative in the presence of the positive expression of *PTEN* by the fibroblasts (internal positive control). (**b**) The SNP6.0 copy number profile shows a focal *PTEN* loss

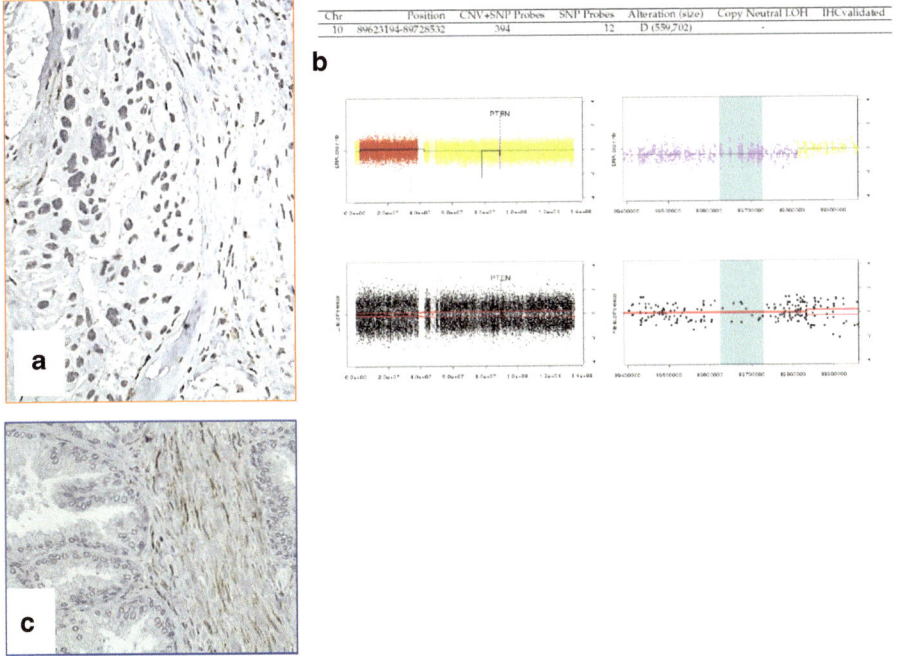

Fig. 2.2 Example of a *PTEN* loss of expression validating a *PTEN* genomic deletion. (**a**) Immunolabeling of *PTEN* protein (clone A2B1, Zymed® laboratories, CA, USA). The metastatic cells are *PTEN* negative in the presence of the positive expression of *PTEN* by the fibroblasts (internal positive control). (**b**) The SNP6.0 copy number profile shows a focal *PTEN* deletion. (**c**) The external positive control represented by the intracytoplasmic positivity of the normal prostatic fibroblasts

2.5 Conclusion and Challenges

Every step of the patient's management in the context of precision medicine requires the pathologist expertise. Before genomic analyses, the pathologist has the key role to diagnose the metastatic disease and to enrich the sample that will be submitted for DNA extraction with tumor cells. After genomic analyses, the pathologist helps to confirm the molecular alterations such as *PTEN* losses in order to facilitate the therapeutic decision.

Pathologist's challenges for the future will be to standardize the management of small samples submitted for diagnosis even those obtained from routine diagnostic activity in order to provide high-quality nucleic acids from formalin-fixed paraffin-embedded tumor tissues. The pathologist will have to sort and to enrich either in tumor cells or in tumor stromal cells the material provided for molecular analyses.

Subsequently, after molecular analyses, the pathologists have to improve simultaneous in situ analyses of several proteins expression in tumor tissues. With the geneticists, they will have to provide comprehensive and straightforward diagnosis reports that integrate the in situ expression data together with the molecular data, in a way suitable for clinical practice.

The pathologists also provide fresh samples of the metastatic tissue for xenografts that will probably play in the near future a key role in assessing tumor sensitivity to selected targeted therapies.

Reference

Le Tourneau C, Mitry E, Goncalves A et al (2014) Randomized phase II trial comparing therapy based on tumor molecular profiling versus conventional therapy in patients with refractory cancer: results of the feasibility part of the SHIVA trial. Br J Cancer 111:17–24

Chapter 3
Basis for Molecular Genetics in Cancer

Gaëlle Pierron

3.1 Introduction

Tumors used to be classified with clinical, radiological, and pathological criteria based on their specific morphological aspects. Consequently, current therapeutic decisions in oncology are strongly influenced by histology rather than by molecular or genomic aberrations. Nevertheless, most cancer genomes undergo genomic instability, which is responsible for the wide repertoire of chromosomal aberrations. Certain chromosomal aberrations are functionally important to the initiation and growth of cancer (drivers), while others merely represent random somatic changes that carry no selective advantage to the cancer cell but can impact stromal interaction or cellular differentiation (passengers). The increasing knowledge and characterization of these molecular changes allowed by the advances in molecular biology and/or high-throughput sequencing techniques inaugurated the integration of genomic information into disease classification leading to molecular pathology.

This comprehensive approach integrating morphological, molecular, and genomic information is currently changing cancer diagnostics: disease classification may be improved by the characterization of somatic genomic alterations acquired during carcinogenesis. Prediction of effective and selective therapies can be wisely chosen according to oncogenic driver lesions considered as therapeutic targets. Moreover and from a global point of view, signaling pathways affected by genomic alterations may be used as prognostic parameters to predict the need and extent of adjuvant therapy. Genomic profiling is also a useful tool to assess genetic link between primary tumor and its metastasis, or in the case of multiple neoplasia, it allows to observe and document the major alterations conserved and shared or counterselected

G. Pierron
Department of Genetics, Institut Curie, Paris, France
e-mail: Gaelle.pierron@curie.fr

© Springer International Publishing Switzerland 2015
C. Le Tourneau, M. Kamal (eds.), *Pan-cancer Integrative Molecular Portrait Towards a New Paradigm in Precision Medicine*,
DOI 10.1007/978-3-319-22189-2_3

during oncogenesis, highlighting a clonal evolution or subpopulations. Finally, detection and fine characterization of circulating tumor DNA (ctDNA) by mutational profiling may open more widely the field of patient care and follow-up by monitoring the response of tumors to therapy and development of secondary resistance.

Taken together, integrative and comprehensive molecular biopathology closely combined with clinical management of patients show a new path through tumoral heterogeneity and complexity to fight cancer with new approaches, which lay the foundations of precision genomic medicine.

3.2 Genetic Aberrations

The mechanisms that maintain DNA sequences occurring during DNA replication, DNA recombination, or DNA repair are remarkably sophisticated, but they are not error proof and most of the genetic changes could result from failures in the normal mechanisms by which genomes are copied or repaired when damaged and are a testimony of genomic instability. These "mistakes" can lead either to simple changes in DNA sequence, such as the substitution of one base pair by another, or to large-scale chromosomes rearrangements such as losses/deletions, gains/duplications, inversions, and translocations of DNA also called chromosomal instability (CIN). In some cases, DNA level affecting microsatellite (MIN) instability can be seen especially in some colon carcinomas (Lengauer et al. 1998) (Fig. 3.1).

3.2.1 Single-Nucleotide Variation (SNV)

These subtle changes of the genetic sequence, observed at the nucleic level, involve the modification, the deletion, or the insertion of one or few base pairs in the reference sequence. These mutations can appear during the DNA replication or can be

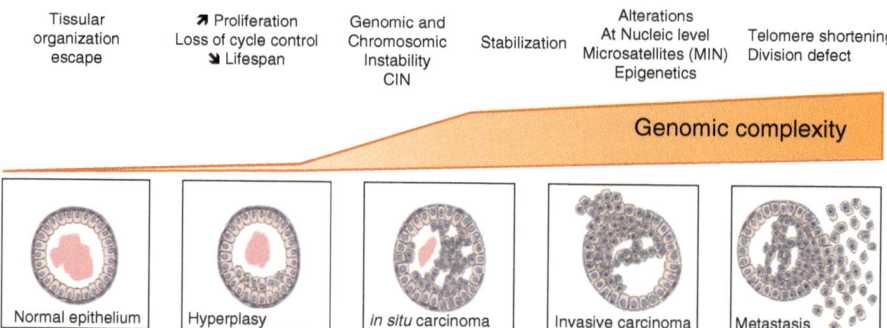

Fig. 3.1 Oncogenesis: Aberration accumulation and genomic complexity

caused by exogenous (X-rays, UV, carcinogenic chemical substances, etc.) or endogenous (free radicals produced during metabolism, etc.) agents.

From a chemical point of view, there are two types of point mutations: transition mutations and transversion mutations. Transition mutations occur when a pyrimidine base (i.e., thymine [T] or cytosine [C]) substitutes for another pyrimidine base or when a purine base (i.e., adenine [A] or guanine [G]) substitutes for another purine base, and transversions are a crossing exchange, i.e., a pyrimidine versus a purine and vice versa.

Biologically, three classes of point mutations can be described in addition to small insertions deletions:

- *Silent mutations*
  A silent mutation also called synonymous mutation addresses the same amino acid and has no functional effect on the protein. As 64 codons code only 20 amino acids (degeneracy of the genetic code), a single nucleotide can change, but the new codon specifies the same amino acid.
- *Missense mutations*
  A missense mutation changes a codon in a nonsynonymous manner so that a different amino acid is created. Functionally, these missense point mutations can be conservative or not. For conservative mutations, the properties of the modified amino acid remain the same (hydrophobic, hydrophilic, etc.) whereas for non-conservative ones, the resulting amino acid can confer different properties to the protein. Prediction tools based on physicochemical score assessment usually classify them as "not deleterious" or "tolerant" as they do not seem to have the potential to affect wild-type protein function. The protein may be activated (see the "gain-of-function" section), as illustrated with the *BRAF* p.V600E. This missense mutation changes a valine (codon 600) to glutamic acid and leads to an activation of the *BRAF* protein which causes an unlimited proliferative signaling in cancer cells. Dedicated theranostic approaches can therefore be applied with the use of vemurafenib treatment in mutant V600E-*BRAF* melanoma (Davies et al. 2002; Bollag et al. 2010; Chapman et al. 2011).
- *Nonsense mutations*
  A nonsense mutation converts an amino acid codon into a stop codon (TAA, TAG, TGA), which truncates the protein and impacts its function depending on the position of the stop codon in the frame of the protein.
- *Indels and in-frame or frameshift mutations*
  If the term SNV for single-nucleotide variation is commonly used to describe substitution, it can also be applied to insertions or deletions (indel) of a single or few base pairs.

When the indel is a multiple of three, the consequences are quite simple: a new codon is added or lost, and the neighboring one can also be modified, and even if the sequence is still in frame, it can affect the resulting protein. For example, *EGFR* exon 19 insertions are a family of *EGFR*-tyrosine kinase inhibitors (TKI)-sensitizing mutations, and patients with tumors harboring these mutations should be treated with *EGFR*-TKI (He et al. 2012; Kris et al. 2012).

However, as gene expression is based on the triplet nature of the codons when the indel affects a number of nucleotides that is not divisible by three, the insertion or deletion can change the reading frame, resulting in a completely different translation. The earlier in the sequence the deletion or insertion occurs, the more altered is the protein. The polypeptide being created could be abnormally short (prematured stop codon) or more rarely abnormally long and will most likely be non functional.

3.2.2   Chromosomal Alterations

The study of malignant cells karyotypes showed that the majority of the human cancers had lost and/or won some chromosomal materials also called chromosomal aneuploidy. These losses and gains, often generated by the same kind of mechanisms, can affect all or part of a chromosome, giving rise, respectively, to either numerical or structural chromosomal aberrations. While oncogenic potential of certain aberrations, like translocations or specific amplification, has been demonstrated to be strongly associated with specific cancers and contributes to their formation, other aberrations like large gains or losses appear to be less specific and random, even if in some cancers certain patterns of chromosomal aberrations can be recognized. The understanding of chromosomal aneuploidy and its mechanisms can help improve the knowledge of tumorigenesis (Albertson et al. 2006) (Fig. 3.2).

3.2.2.1   Gains and Losses

Chromosome gains and losses are broad alterations encompassing from few megabases (Mb) to hundred Mb or even whole chromosomes. As these duplications (3–8 copies) or simple deletions (of a unique copy, if the tumor is diploid) are quite large, they can affect hundred of genes and their significance to the carcinogenesis process is less understood. Although there is evidence suggesting chromosome selection preferences for aneuploid cells in certain cancer types and although changes in gene copy number are among the most frequent molecular events in human cancer genome, these kinds of aberrations do not seem to be targetable.

3.2.2.2   Focal Amplifications

Certain tumors present genomic amplifications reflecting the acquisition of an increased number of DNA copies (from 8–10 to hundred sometimes) by multistep processes usually under positive selection. Often associated with late and/or aggressive stages of cancerous progress, these genomic inscreases can be infrachromosomal, and then called HSR for homogeneous staining region, or extrachromosomic as chromosomes double minute, which proposed mechanism is based on "bridge-fusion-break" iterations. Generally associated with the tumoral proliferation, the amplifications can be also found in initial phases in certain sarcomas. These addictions to a number of oncogenic drivers, leading to these amplifications, for example, genomically amplified *MDM2* proteins, *MET*, *HER2*, and *EGFR*, are of particular interest because of pharmacological approaches which can directly target and inhibit the overexpressed protein (Fig. 3.3).

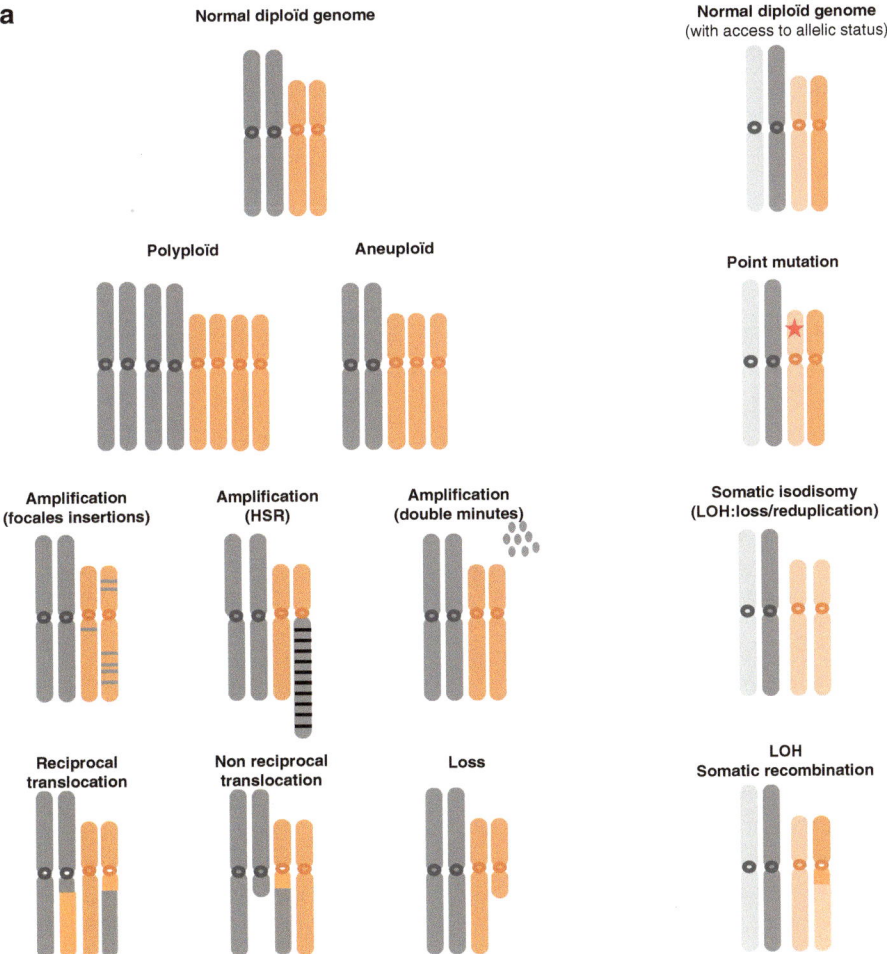

Fig. 3.2 (**a**) Examples of chromosomal alterations, theoretical point of view. (**b**) Examples of chromosomal alterations, chromosomal point of view (Adapted from Albertson et al. 2003)

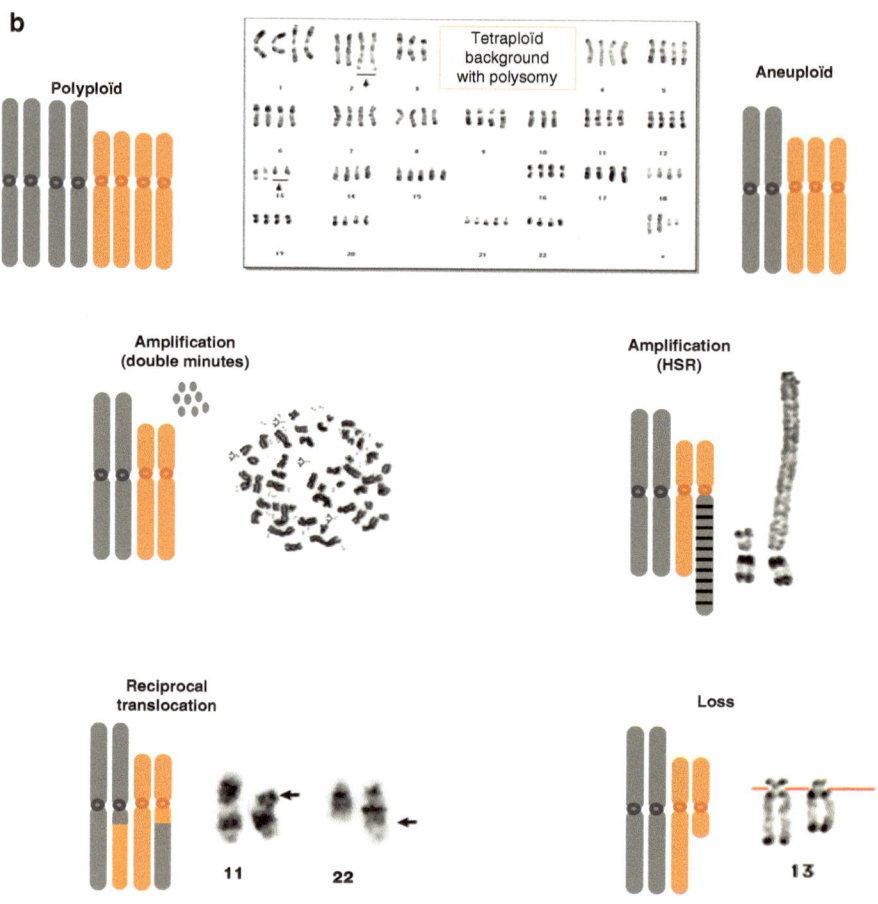

Fig. 3.2 (continued)

3.2.2.3 Homozygous Deletion

In a diploid organism, homozygous deletion refers to the loss of both alleles or a portion of both alleles from a genomic location. By extension, this physical loss affect both copies of the same gene or of the same chromosomal segment of a pair of homologous chromosomes. As multigenic deletion have severe consequences, and as the size of the deleted region is directly correlated to the number of the genes to be lost, the homozygous deletion is often small from few kilobases (Kb), which can arise within a tumor suppressor gene (intragenic deletion) to very few Mb affecting a small number of genes. Losses of *PTEN*, *CDKN2A*, *RB1*, or *SMARCB1* are well-documented examples of genes inactivated by homozygous deletion. The double deleted region can be the intersection of two independent events, two large overlapping deletions (four distinct breakpoints), a small deletion associated to loss

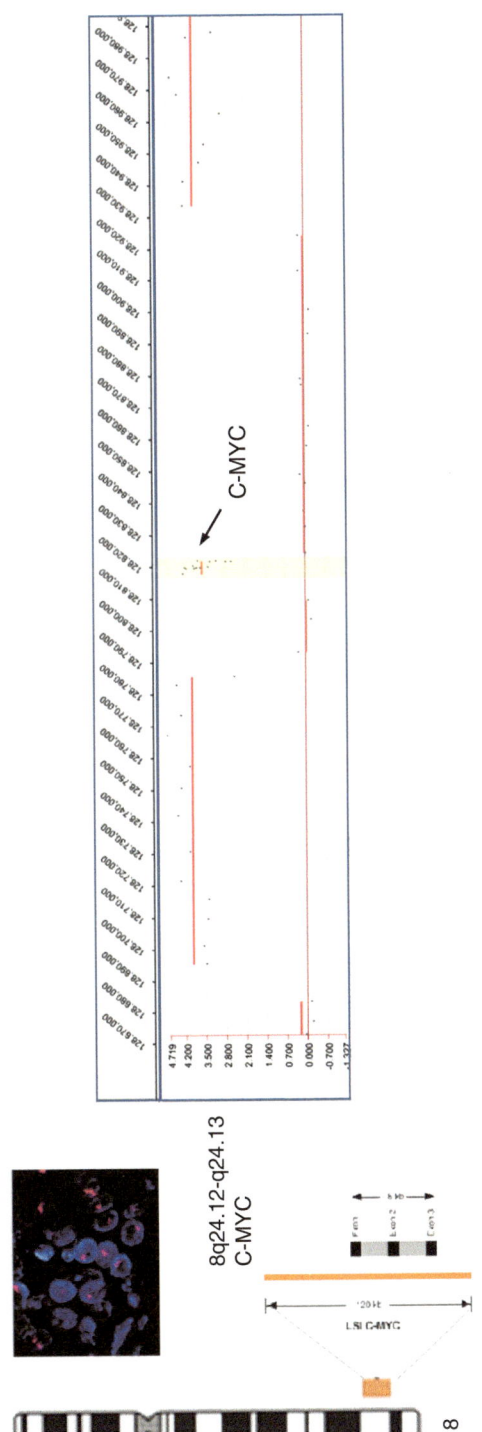

Fig. 3.3 Focal amplification (assessed by FISH and aCGH)

of the whole remaining homologous chromosome (only two different breakpoints on the remaining chromosome), and sometimes a small deletion with loss and reduplication of the chromosome also called somatic isodisomy.

3.2.2.4   Somatic Isodisomy

Isodisomy is a very specific type of genomic aberration in which the two copies of the chromosome originate from the same chromosome (inherited from one parent) with resultant homozygosity at all gene loci on the considered chromosome. Most often, isodisomy concerns an entire chromosome when the homologous chromosome is lost, but it may also be limited to part of a chromosome (segmental isodisomy). The presence of isodisomy in a tumor genome can highlight a simple mechanism to obtain biallelic inactivation of a tumor suppressor gene which is already mutated or disrupted on one allele (Fig. 3.4).

3.2.2.5   Structural Aberration

As translocations directly affect a small number of genes, the role of many translocations in cancer causation has become much clearer over the years. These translocations can be within a chromosome (with the homologous chromosome or inversion inside the same chromosome). They can also occur between different chromosomes and in a nonreciprocal manner (often with loss of material) or can form ring chromosome.

3.2.2.6   Recurring Translocations

In 1960, studying chronic myeloid leukemia, Nowell and Hungerford observed the first cytogenetic reorganization acquired and recurring: the Philadelphia chromosome. This recombination between chromosomes 9 and 22 leads to the translocation t(9;22)(q34;q11) (Nowell and Hungerford 1960).

These chromosome translocations can have two types of consequences:

- Upregulation of the expression of a gene. In this case, the reorganization juxtaposes the strong elements of regulation of the promoter of one a gene (like IgH or TCR) near an oncogene and increases its transcription (Ott et al. 2013).The mechanism is particularly frequent in lymphoid malignancies, with the first studied example: the t(8;14)(q24;32) in Burkitt's lymphoma. These translocations are mostly generated during V(D)J recombination.
- Breakpoints formation of a fusion gene transcript appears to leukemia (CML) breakpoints on each chromosome occur in two genes leading to the formation of a fusion gene with new and oncogenic properties. The resulting fusion transcript appears to be highly specific like *BCR-ABL* in chronic myelogenous leukemia (CML).

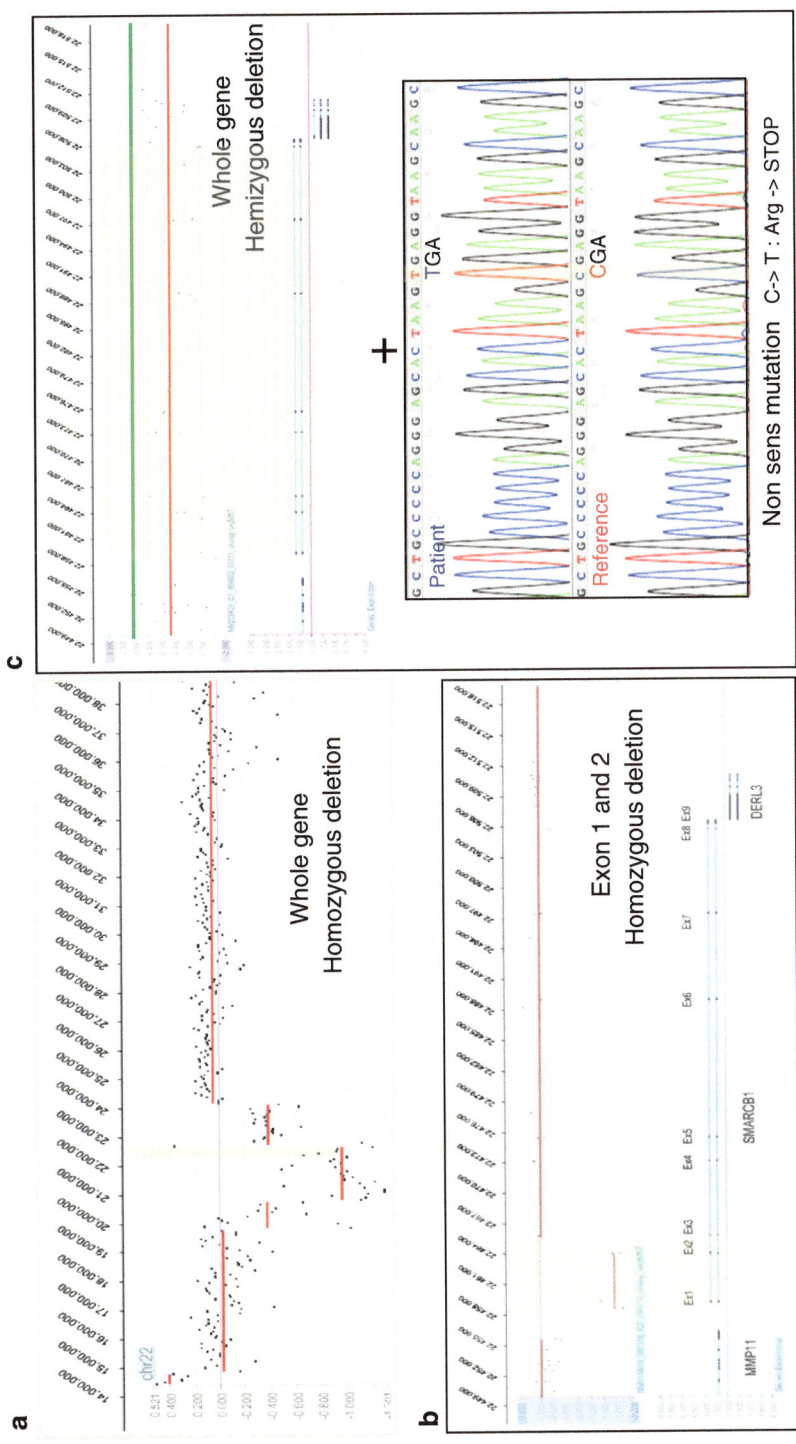

Fig. 3.4 Biallelic inactivation. (**a**) Whole-gene homozygous deletion (aCGH); (**b**) focal homozygous deletion within a gene (aCGH); (**c**) hemizygous deletion associated with nonsense point mutation (aCGH + Sanger sequencing)

The identification of fusion transcripts not only supports the diagnosis but provides the basis for the development of novel therapeutic strategies aimed at blocking the aberrant activity of chimeric proteins. Molecular biology and, in particular, cytogenetic and qualitative and quantitative RT-PCR technologies allow with high efficiency and specificity the determination of specific fusion transcripts resulting from chromosomal translocations. In prostate cancer, the TMPRSS2-ERG fusion is found in ~50 % of all tumors, making it the single most common genetic lesion of this disease (Gopalan et al. 2009). In Ewing's sarcoma (EWSR1-ETS) or alveolar rhabdomyosarcomas (PAX3/7-FOXO1), the fusion detection as specific marker is mandatory for molecular diagnosis.

3.2.2.7   Chromothripsis

The recent discovery of a new kind of massive chromosomal rearrangement in different cancers, named "*chromothripsis*" (*chromo* for chromosome, *thripsis* for shattering), has questioned the established models for a progressive development of tumors. Indeed, this phenomenon, which is characterized by the shattering of one or a few chromosome segments followed by a random reassembly of the fragments generated, occurs during one unique cellular event. Diverse situations can cause chromothripsis (radiations, telomere erosion, abortive apoptosis, etc.), and two express "repair routes" are used by the cell to chaotically reorganize the chromosomal regions concerned: nonhomologous end joining and repair by replicative stress (Korbel and Campbell 2013; Zhang et al. 2013)

3.2.3   Cancer Genes

Through the years, the definitions of the genes involved in cancers did not stop evolving. Historically, these were highlighted by their capacities to transform normal cells (discovery of c-Src via v-Src in Rous's sarcoma) (Rous and Robertson 1917; Stehelin et al. 1976) or to revert a so-called "malignant" phenotype once introduced into cultured cells (experiments of somatic hybrids) (Ephrussi et al. 1969).

They were then characterized by the type and/or the number of mutation conferring them their tumoral abilities, but at the moment, their classification refers much more to their function and the modification of this one in the tumoral context. Thus, two big categories of genes involved in cancer can globally be defined: those whose alterations cause a gain of function and those whose aberrations lead to a loss of function.

3.2.3.1   "Gain-of-Function (GoF)" Genes

In their normal nonmutated state, GoF genes are called proto-oncogenes and are directly or indirectly involved in controlling the rate of cell growth and are implicated in the regulation of cell division. When altered by a genetic event, such as point mutation, translocation, or chromosome amplification, these cancer-promoting genes become then abnormally activated and named oncogenes.

Mutations affecting oncogenes are most often somatic, but germinal activating mutations have already been described (e.g. *RET* involved in multiple endocrine tumor type II and *MET* gene in hereditary papillary cancer of the kidney) (Santoro et al. 2002; Linehan et al. 2007).

The activation of GoF is dominant, the alteration of only one allele being sufficient to confer an oncogenic potential. The consequences of this activation can be seen at the expression level or at the DNA level of the targeted gene.

Examples of Gain-of-Function Mechanisms

The increase of the transcription of an oncogene can result from the translocation in its closeness of strong sequences of regulation (promoting sequences), which change the modulation of the native level of expression leading to an overexpression, like c-*MYC* in the t(8;14) translocation arising in Burkitt's lymphoma. The mutation affecting the nucleotidic structure of an oncogene led to the synthesis of a functionally abnormal protein. So fusion genes resulting of chromosomes translocation can produce chimeric proteins such as *BCR-ABL* (Philadelphia chromosome marker) in chronic myeloid leukemia or truncated protein like *NOTCH* in lymphoblastic leukemia (Grabher et al. 2006). Lastly, point mutations can also drive the synthesis of proteins blocked in active configuration (like for *K-RAS CTNNB1* (beta-catenin) (Eser et al. 2014) (Rosenbluh et al. 2014)), and focal oncogene amplifications are classical mechanisms of gain of function (like for *CDK4* or *MDM2*).

Whatever the mechanisms of activation of a "proto-oncogene," its overexpression or maintained expression is often connected to a process of differentiation, proliferation, or cellular survival and consequently drives tumorigenesis.

3.2.3.2 "Loss-of-Function (LoF)" Genes

Historically, only genes matching with the model of Knudson (Knudson 1971, 1993) were qualified as loss-of-function genes. In this model, the so-called "two-hit model", the genetic inactivation (germinal and/or somatic) of both alleles of the gene is mandatory to drive the tumoral development. The study of the somatic hybrids (merging normal cells and tumoral cells) allowed to highlight the reversion of the tumoral phenotype associated with this loss of function, by the addition of a wild-type copy of the gene of interest (Ephrussi et al. 1969). These genes were then qualified as tumor suppressor genes (TSG). Since then, the study of the function of the genes inactivated in the cancerous processes, like control of cell proliferation or maintenance of the integrity of the cellular genetic material, had highlighted new definitions for TSG which can be subclassified in gatekeepers, caretakers, or landscapers (Kinzler and Vogelstein 1996; Kinzler et al. 1998; Macleod 2000).

3.2.3.3 Gatekeepers

Gatekeepers are genes encoding proteins that regulate cell proliferation. They act as "guardians" that prevent cells from passing through cell cycle checkpoints by countering the progression of cellular growth and encouraging apoptosis. Thus, their inactivation allows cells to bypass the cell cycle checkpoints, leading to unrestricted proliferation, differentiation, and immortality of tumor cells. Alteration of one copy (allele) of a gatekeeper gene predisposes an individual to cancer, while mutation of the two alleles often leads to neoplasia. Well-known gatekeeper genes are, for (He et al. 1997) example, *RB1, BRCA1, CDKN2A,* and *APC.*

3.2.3.4 Caretakers

Caretaker genes, a second type of tumor suppressor gene, maintain and protect the integrity of the genome and may sometimes be referred to as "genome maintenance genes." In general, these genes are involved in genome stability, via DNA repair, and help prevent accumulation of mutations in gatekeeper genes or oncogenes. Caretaker mechanisms include DNA base excision repair, nucleotide excision repair, prevention of oncogenic chromosomal rearrangement, nonhomologous end joining, mismatched repair, and telomere maintenance. Two examples are *MLH1/MSH2*, which are involved in DNA mismatch repair, and XP-A, which is involved in the nucleotide excision repair pathway (Parsons et al. 2012; Ding et al. 2012; Epstein 2013).

A faulty protein arising from a mutant caretaker gene can lead to certain genomic instabilities such as microsatellites, point mutations, or chromosomal instabilities, and then, affected cells easily accumulate mutations due to impaired genome maintenance.

3.2.3.5 Other Functions and Overlaps Between Gatekeepers and Caretakers

In addition to their anticancer functions, gatekeeper and caretaker genes have been known to have an effect on senescence, especially later in life. Gatekeepers may induce aging, and caretakers are known to maintain telomeres. Dysfunctional gatekeepers and caretakers may thus lead not only to cancer but also to premature aging. Some genes such as *TP53* falls into both categories. *TP53* is most often identified as a gatekeeper, since it is directly involved in cell cycle regulation and cellular proliferation. However, *TP53* also has many caretaker functions and is involved in DNA repair mechanisms (Soussi and Wiman 2015)

3.2.3.6 Landscapers

Recently, a third group of tumor suppressor genes has been proposed. These are called "landscaper genes," and they encode products that help create environments that control cell growth. Landscapers were first discovered when lesions were found in cells surrounding tumor tissue in juvenile polyposis syndrome. It was observed that the initiating lesions occurred not in the tumor cells, but rather in the surrounding stromal cells. Without functional copies of a landscaper gene, the microenvironment may become abnormal such that it promotes transformation of normal epithelial cells. Predicted mechanisms involving these landscaper genes include the regulation of extracellular matrix proteins, cellular surface markers, cellular adhesion molecules, and growth factors. One possibility is that mutants in landscapers involved in regulating cell membranes may trigger chemokine release, leading to unregulated cellular proliferation. An example of a landscaper gene is *PTEN*. Sometimes LoF genes can have multiple functions according to their tissue localization, such as *NF1* which acts as gatekeeper in Schwann's cells, and play a role landscaper on fibroblasts composing the tumor (Macleod 2000).

Examples of Loss-of-Function Mechanisms

Genetic mechanisms driving to the loss of function of a gene suppressor of tumors are varied. Arising at the nucleotidic or chromosome level, they can involve point mutation and losses of genetic material by interstitial deletion, by loss of arm or whole chromosome, by unbalanced translocations, or passages in the homozygosity by mitotic recombination or chromosome loss followed by reduplication (isodisomy) (see Part I).

But the analysis of experimental models in mice inactivated for one allele of a TSG did not still highlight the deletion or the alteration of the second allele (Yamasaki et al. 1996; Zhu et al. 1998). Furthermore, the exhaustive analysis of certain recurring deletions in human tumors did not allowed to identify a gene answering in classic criteria of biallelic inactivation of TSG. Other mechanisms were thus proposed:

* *The epigenetic inactivation*
  These genetic changes do not affect the DNA itself but modify nevertheless in a hereditary way the activity of the targeted genes. The involved mechanisms can include stable feedback loops, nuclear sequestration, differential replication timing, acquisition of inherited structures of the chromatin, or most of the time cytosine methylation localized in 5′ by a dinucleotide CpG island (Fruhwald et al. 2002). The hypermethylation of regions promoters of key genes is much better characterized in human cancers and is associated with an inappropriate repression of the targeted genes. More and more candidate TSG seems to present hypermethylations of their promoter which participate in their inactivation, as in the case of *CDKN2B* (Herman et al. 1997) or *MGMT* (Esteller et al. 2000).
  Hypermethylation and other epigenetic mechanisms can be considered as real mutational events. Often secondary when they are associated to deletions or losses of heterozygosity, these mechanisms can also arise alone and prematurely. They can participate in steps of genetic inactivation which sometimes is enough to confer a selective advantage essential to the tumoral evolution.

- *The haploinsufficiency*
  When the genetic aberration affects a gene, the product of which has to be tightly controlled since the slightest imbalance in the rate of production can lead to a major phenotype. This hypothesis was confirmed in murine models inactivated for only one allele of various TSG like p27/Kip1, Dmp1, Pten (Inoue et al. 2001; Quon and Berns 2001). The protein regulates negatively the activation of AKT kinases (Stambolic et al. 1998). The haploid expression of *PTEN* is not enough to fulfill its function, allowing the activation of a significant level of AKT which can block the apoptosis inferred by FAS (Di Cristofano et al. 1999). The haploinsufficiency of the TSG seems to present diverse degrees of consequences on the physiology of the cell. The inactivation of the first allele would favor a clonal expansion and would so increase the probability of a second event to arise (Cook and McCaw 2000).
- *The dominant negative mutations*
  Both frequent and contradictory mechanisms with the recessive character of a TSG can be observed when inactivating mutations occur in proteins belonging to multimeric complexes. For example, these proteins can be for *TP53*, when mutated, more stable than the wild-type protein with a longer half-life (William et al. 2012) or for PPARgamma (R288H in colon cancer) can retain a total or partial ligand binding domain but lose the ability to activate transcription (Sarraf et al. 1999). The change is then codominant.

3.3   Conclusions

Tumorigenesis requires the acquisition by the cell of essential physiological skills which reflect its genetic abnormalities. The study of these multiple genetic aberrations, which can arise either at chromosome level or at nucleotidic level in key genes (oncogene or tumor suppressor gene), is then mandatory to a proper and integrative understanding of tumorigenic process.

   To be able to properly integrate and stratify these aberrations in a smart algorithm, each kind of point mutations, translocations, deletions, or amplifications has to be detected with high specificity and sensibility. Many technological choices are available. So, regarding the technology efficiency and the experiment cost (in terms of biological material and funds), a process combining NGS (dedicated panel, WES, WGS), genome-wide aCGH, and IHC validation, seems to be the most relevant choice.

   Finally, the analysis of somatic aberrations must also take into account that deciphering genetic aberration in tumor cells can be sometimes a real challenge because the sample is not always composed of 100 % of tumor cells (stromal contamination, lymphoid infiltration, etc.). In addition, tumor cells can be tri- or tetraploid. Consequently, the interpretation of the observed aberrations has to be set on solid oncogenetic backgrounds and has to integrate all these parameters.

References

Albertson DG, Collins C, McCormick F, Gray JW. (2003). Chromosome aberrations in solid tumors.Nat Genet. 34(4):369–376.

Albertson DG, Snijders AM, Fridlyand J et al (2006) Genomic analysis of tumors by array comparative genomic hybridization: more is better. Cancer Res 66(7):3955–3956

Bollag G, Hirth P, Tsai J et al (2010) Clinical efficacy of a RAF inhibitor needs broad target blockade in *BRAF* mutant melanoma. Nature 467(7315):596–599

Chapman PB, Hauschild A, Robert C et al (2011) Improved survival with vemurafenib in melanoma with *BRAF* V600E mutation. N Engl J Med 364(26):2507–2516

Cook WD, McCaw BJ (2000) Accommodating haploinsufficient tumor suppressor genes in Knudson's model. Oncogene 19(30):3434–3438

Davies H, Bignell GR, Cox C et al (2002) Mutations of the *BRAF* gene in human cancer. Nature 417(6892):949–954

Di Cristofano A, Kotsi P, Peng YF et al (1999) Impaired Fas response and autoimmunity in Pten+/– mice. Science 285(5436):2122–2125

Ding D, Zhang Y, Yu H et al (2012) Genetic variation of XPA gene and risk of cancer: a systematic review and pooled analysis. Int J Cancer 131(2):488–496

Ephrussi B, Davidson RL, Weiss MC (1969) Malignancy of somatic cell hybrids. Nature 224(5226):1314–1316

Epstein RJ (2013) The unpluggable in pursuit of the undruggable: tackling the dark matter of the cancer therapeutics universe. Front Oncol 3:304

Eser S, Schnieke A, Schneider G et al (2014) Oncogenic *KRAS* signalling in pancreatic cancer. Br J Cancer 111(5):817–822

Esteller M, Garcia-Foncillas J, Andion E et al (2000) Inactivation of the DNA-repair gene MGMT and the clinical response of gliomas to alkylating agents. N Engl J Med 343(19):1350–1354

Freed-Pastor WA, Prives C. (2012) Mutant p53: one name, many proteins. Genes Dev. Jun 15;26(12):1268–86.

Fruhwald S, Herk E, Petnehazy T et al (2002) Sufentanil potentiates the inhibitory effect of epinephrine on intestinal motility. Intensive Care Med 28(1):74–80

Gopalan A, Leversha MA, Satagopan JM et al (2009) TMPRSS2-ERG gene fusion is not associated with outcome in patients treated by prostatectomy. Cancer Res 69(4):1400–1406

Grabher C, von Boehmer H, Look AT (2006) Notch 1 activation in the molecular pathogenesis of T-cell acute lymphoblastic leukaemia. Nat Rev Cancer 6(5):347–359

Hanahan D, Weinberg RA (2000) The hallmarks of cancer. Cell 100(1):57–70

Hanahan D, Weinberg RA (2011) Hallmarks of cancer: the next generation. Cell 144(5):646–674

He M, Capelletti M, Nafa K et al (1997) Distinct patterns of inactivation of p15INK4B and p16INK4A characterize the major types of hematological malignancies. Cancer Res 57(5):837–841

He M, Capelletti M, Nafa K, Yun CH, Arcila ME, Miller VA, Ginsberg MS, Zhao B, Kris MG, Eck MJ, Jänne PA, Ladanyi M, Oxnard GR. (2012) *EGFR* exon 19 insertions: a new family of sensitizing *EGFR* mutations in lung adenocarcinoma. Clin Cancer Res 15;18(6):1790–1797.

Herman JG, Civin CI, Issa JP, Collector MI, Sharkis SJ, Baylin SB. (1997) Distinct patterns of inactivation of p15INK4B and p16INK4A characterize the major types of hematological malignancies. Cancer Res. Mar 1;57(5):837–41.

Huang FW, Hodis E, Xu MJ et al (2013) Highly recurrent TERT promoter mutations in human melanoma. Science 339(6122):957–959

Inoue K, Zindy F, Randle DH et al (2001) Dmp1 is haplo-insufficient for tumor suppression and modifies the frequencies of Arf and p53 mutations in Myc-induced lymphomas. Genes Dev 15(22):2934–2939

Kinzler KW, Vogelstein B (1996) Lessons from hereditary colorectal cancer. Cell 87(2):159–170

Kinzler KW, Vogelstein B. (1998) Landscaping the cancer terrain. Science. May 15;280(5366):1036–7

Knudson AG Jr. Mutation and cancer: statistical study of retinoblastoma. (1971) Proc Natl Acad Sci USA. Apr;68(4):820–3.

Knudson AG. (1993). Antioncogenes and human cancer. Proc Natl Acad Sci USA. Dec 1;90(23):10914–21.

Korbel JO, Campbell PJ (2013) Criteria for inference of chromothripsis in cancer genomes. Cell 152(6):1226–1236

Kris MG, Eck MJ, Jänne PA et al (2012) *EGFR* exon 19 insertions: a new family of sensitizing *EGFR* mutations in lung adenocarcinoma. Clin Cancer Res 18(6):1790–1797

Lengauer C, Kinzler KW, Vogelstein B (1998) Genetic instabilities in human cancers. Nature 396(6712):643–649

Linehan WM, Pinto PA, Srinivasan R et al (2007) Identification of the genes for kidney cancer: opportunity for disease-specific targeted therapeutics. Clin Cancer Res 13(2 Pt 2):671s–679s

Macleod K (2000) Tumor suppressor genes. Curr Opin Genet Dev 10(1):81–93

Nowell PC, Hungerford DA (1960) Chromosome studies on normal and leukemic human leukocytes. J Natl Cancer Inst 25:85–109

Ott G, Rosenwald A, Campo E (2013) Understanding MYC-driven aggressive B-cell lymphomas: pathogenesis and classification. Blood 122(24):3884–3891

Parsons MT, Buchanan DD, Thompson B et al (2012) Correlation of tumour *BRAF* mutations and *MLH1* methylation with germline mismatch repair (MMR) gene mutation status: a literature review assessing utility of tumour features for MMR variant classification. J Med Genet 49(3):151–157

Quon KC, Berns A (2001) Haplo-insufficiency? Let me count the ways. Genes Dev 15(22): 2917–2921

Rosenbluh J, Wang X, Hahn WC (2014) Genomic insights into WNT/β-catenin signaling. Trends Pharmacol Sci 35(2):103–109

Rous P, Robertson OH (1917) The normal fate of erythrocytes: I. the findings in healthy animals. J Exp Med 25(5):651–663

Santoro M, Melillo RM, Carlomagno F et al (2002) Molecular mechanisms of RET activation in human cancer. Ann N Y Acad Sci 963:116–21

Sarraf P, Mueller E, Smith WM et al (1999) Loss-of-function mutations in PPAR gamma associated with human colon cancer. Mol Cell 3(6):799–804

Soussi T, Wiman KG (2015) *TP53*: an oncogene in disguise. Cell Death Differ. doi:10.1038/cdd.2015.53

Stambolic V, Suzuki A, de la Pompa JL et al (1998) Negative regulation of PKB/Akt-dependent cell survival by the tumor suppressor *PTEN*. Cell 95(1):29–39

Stehelin D, Varmus HE, Bishop JM et al (1976) DNA related to the transforming gene(s) of avian sarcoma viruses is present in normal avian DNA. Nature 260(5547):170–173

Wood LD, Parsons DW, Jones S et al (2007) The genomic landscapes of human breast and colorectal cancers. Science 318(5853):1108–1113

Yamasaki H, Krutovskikh V, Mesnil M et al (1996) Connexin genes and cell growth control. Arch Toxicol Suppl 18:105–114

Zhang CZ, Leibowitz ML, Pellman D (2013) Chromothripsis and beyond: rapid genome evolution from complex chromosomal rearrangements. Genes Dev 27(23):2513–2530

Zhu JJ, Santarius T, Wu X, Tsong J, Guha A, Wu JK, Hudson TJ, Black PM. (1998) Screening for loss of heterozygosity and microsatellite instability in oligodendrogliomas. Genes Chromosomes Cancer. Mar;21(3):207–16.

Chapter 4
Microarrays-Based Molecular Profiling to Identify Genomic Alterations

David Gentien and Cecile Reyes

4.1 Introduction

First genomic portraits have been made when the setup of karyotype was achieved in the middle of the twentieth century (Ferguson-Smith 2008). At this time, the number of chromosome, the size of chromosome, the localization of centrosome relative to entire chromosome, and the number and the position of condensed chromatin (heterochromatin) *versus* unpacked chromatin (euchromatin) were the hallmarks of genome stability. Even if the first chromosomes were observed in 1842 by Carl Wilhelm on plants, another German, anatomo-pathologist Waldeyer used the name of chromosome in 1888 when he described the mitotic process. Decades of investigations were necessary to fix the correct number of chromosomes in human cells (Harper 2006) and to reveal that the cytogenetics of a normal diploid organism contains 46 chromosomes in human somatic cells, or 23 in human germline cells. Protocols of chromosome spreads' staining based on fixation of Giemsa onto GC rich were set up to distinguished chromosomes and to identify G and R bands. By chance different profiles of positive and negative brands were obtained per chromosome, providing one of the first genomic maps. The numbers of bands were useful for chromosome identification. The number of chromosomes was set as a marker to evaluate genome ploidy, and the position and size of bands were useful to identify DNA deletion, inversion, and translocation. One of the limitations of karyotyping and chromosome banding is the number of distinguished bands obtained depending on the stage of condensation of the chromatin (metaphase or mid-prophase). The number of bands gives the resolution of the analysis, for example, 350 bands could

D. Gentien (✉) • C. Reyes
Translational Research Department, Institut Curie, Paris, France
e-mail: david.gentien@curie.fr; cecile.reyes@curie.fr

© Springer International Publishing Switzerland 2015
C. Le Tourneau, M. Kamal (eds.), *Pan-cancer Integrative Molecular Portrait Towards a New Paradigm in Precision Medicine*,
DOI 10.1007/978-3-319-22189-2_4

be detected in metaphase given a low resolution (7–10 Mb/band), or 1250–2000 bands could be detected in mid-prophase given a high resolution (1.5 Mb/band) for a human genome (Bickmore 2001, Fig. 4.1). Bands are counted from the centromeres and labeled with a specific name containing the chromosome number and a letter specific to the arm (long/q, short/p) and the number of the band.

The karyotyping analysis, tool for cytogenetics, was useful for human genetic research (i.e., species evolutionary mitosis and meiotic processes etc.) and in medicine to associate genomic disorders to clinics (translocation, leukemia; gains, Huntington disease, trisomy 21 in Down syndrome; sex chromosomal aberrations, Turner syndrome; etc.). Interestingly, such techniques open new area of research such as DNA replication, and gene dosage theories appeared to be linked to chromosome copy numbers. In 1961, Mary Lyon proposed that X chromosome compaction was related to the random inactivation of one female X chromosome.

Main biochemical discoveries made in 1950s such as the understanding of the DNA composition specificity (A, T, C, and G) demonstrated by E. Chargaff, the characterization of the DNA structure made by J. Watson and F. Crick in 1953, and the genetic code leading to a specific protein synthesis done by M. Nirenberg in 1963 solved basic issues in biology. In 1977, a rapid sequencing approach was described by F. Sanger using labeled and degenerated nucleotides (dideoxynucleo-

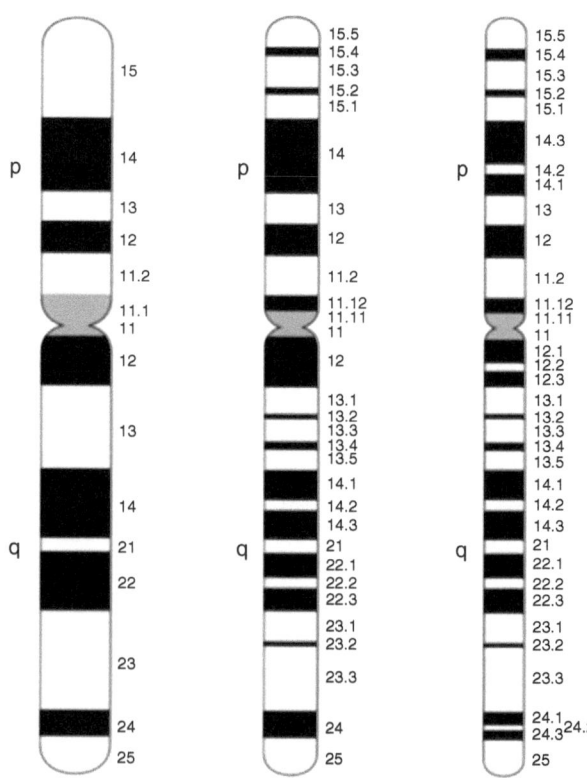

Fig. 4.1 G band ideograms of human chromosome 11 at (*from left to right*) 350, 550, and 850 band resolution (From Bickmore 2001)

tide) to synthesize a new DNA strand that migrates into an acrylamide gel according to their size, upon an electric field (electrophoresis). In 1983, a reaction called polymerase chain reaction (PCR) was set up by K. Mullis to amplify a portion of a genome producing billion copies of a target in 4 hours.

Those two techniques were very helpful to imagine in 1985 the sequencing of the human genome and launch the international programs such as the Human Genome Project, which began in 1990 in the USA, the UK, France, Germany, Japan (NIH, Welcome Trust Sanger Center, etc.). In the summer 2000, a public consortia and a private company (Celera, headed by Craig Venter) proposed a first draft of the human genome, revealing that 95 % of the genome was sequenced and also that two human genomes are 99.5 % identical and contain ~30,000 genes in a ~3 Gb. This was possible using cloning methods inserting long genomic fragments (~200,000 bp) into bacteria to create libraries, followed by sub-libraries containing smaller pieces of DNA (1000–2000 bp), which were used for sequencing and mapping.

In the other hand, the HapMap Project (International HapMap Consortium 2003, Japan, the UK, Canada, China, Nigeria, and the USA) analyzes thousands of genomes to identify sequence variants across multiple populations (Asian, African, Europe, etc.) that would affect common or specific disease. As ten millions of single nucleotide polymorphisms (SNPs) may occur in the human genome, the way to analyze SNP consists to genotype each allele. The analysis of SNP shared by several DNA was useful to identify common region, inherited, for example, in order to reduce the number of interesting SNP into haplotypes. The map of haplotypes was predicted to contain SNP present in 90 % of population, and they were evaluated by sequencing the targeted SNP (in the HapMap programs). Several tools were designed to analyze thousands of SNPs, randomly speared among the genome or not. The interest in such study is to perform linkage study that facilitates the understanding of a specific disease mutation. It is interesting to know if a specific population is affected or not by a mutation and if it is due to a specific haplotype or SNP. This information could be also taken into account to adjust treatment or avoid side effects (e.g., metabolism of a drug).

4.2 Fluorescence In Situ Hybridization Techniques

In order to analyze more precisely the number of chromosomes and their content, in situ hybridization techniques were developed on metaphases or on fixed tissue sections, to hybridize onto nucleic acids, single-strand DNA or RNA molecules coupled to a radioactive, and fluorescent probe or non-fluorescent probes (i.e., biotin). In the late 1960s, rough first protocols were set up to identify, for example, the localization of amplified ribosomal genes in *Xenopus* oocytes, by the use of purified and radioactive ribosomal RNA in 1969 (John et al. 1969; Gall and Pardue 1969; Langer-Safer et al. 1982). From the 1980s till date, hundreds of publications describe easier methods to prepare probes by genetic engineering coupled to specific fluorescent probes in order to detect loci copy numbers (Volpi and Bridger 2008). Most of the probes used for fluorescent in situ hybridization (FISH) approaches today were generated in the Human Genome Project.

Depending on the aim of the FISH, the probes used can be short (10–25 nt) to detect messenger RNA or microRNA, for example, or longer to detect repetitive sequences near centromeres such as satellite DNA, telomeres, or other sequences of interest. Multiprobes can be applied for translocation assessments or for the quantification of repetitive elements or transposons (Singer 1982; Weiner 2002) such as SINE (Short Interspersed Nuclear Elements) or LINE (Long Interspersed Nuclear elements). Furthermore, multicolor FISH techniques were used to perform chromosome painting (Ried et al. 1998, Fig. 4.2), in order to monitor rearrangement in long genes such as large rearrangements of *BRCA1* or BRCA2 in breast and ovarian cancers (Gad et al. 2001, 2002).

In breast cancers, human epidermal growth factor receptor 2 (Her2) is quantified in routine on fixed tissues. The receptor is detected using dedicated antibodies to perform immunochemistry (IHC). When the IHC results are equivocal, the FISH technique is used to confirm the Her2 status. Specific probes for Her2 hybridize a 190 kb region (17q11.2-q12) including the Her2 gene (i.e., PathVysion Her2 Kit, FDA approved, Abbott Molecular). Furthermore, in order to take into account polysomy, another probe located in the centromere of chromosome 17 is also hybridized on centromeric alpha satellite sequences (CEP17 (Waye and Willard 1986)). This second probe is labeled with a different fluorescent probe. Almost 20 metaphases should be analyzed to quantify the number of Her2 and CEP17 genomic copies. Depending on the number of Her2 copy number (>2, ≥4, >6) and depending on the Her2/Cep17 ratio (<2), the result will indicate positive or negative status and may orient patient into Her2-targeted therapies (http://www.asco.org/guidelines/her2).

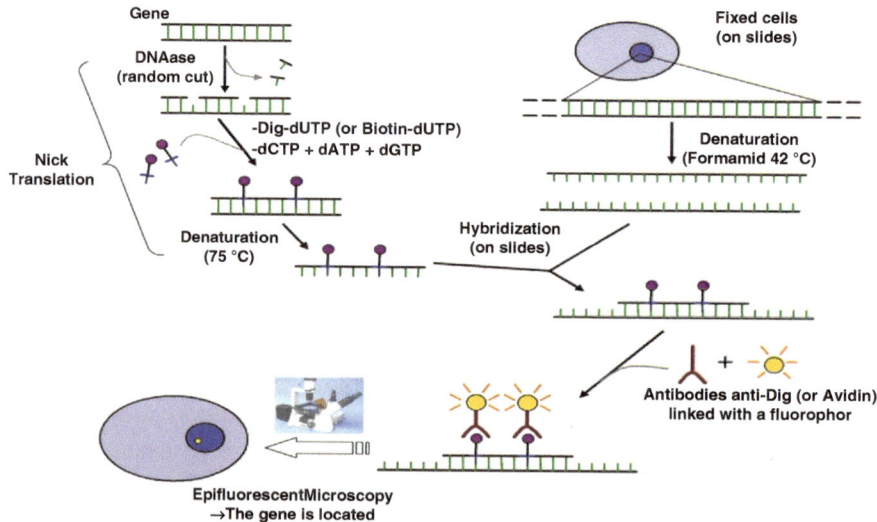

Fig. 4.2 Principle of fluorescent in situ hybridization (FISH)

4.3 Comparative Genomic Hybridization

Comparative genomic hybridization (CGH) appeared in 1992 (Kallioniemi et al. 1992) to improve resolution of karyotyping and FISH techniques. CGH technique allows to gain in resolution of karyotypes as compared to Giemsa banding to enlarge the number of analyzed targets as compared to the FISH technique. CGH techniques identify more precisely genomic aberrations such as losses, deletions, gains, amplification, and certain translocation. To perform a CGH, high-quality normal metaphase spreads needed to be spread on a glass slide from normal cells (Fig. 4.3). Next two different labeled DNAs are hybridized on the slide under specific conditions (Weiss et al. 1999) to avoid nonspecific hybridization of DNA onto repetitive sequences (addition of human Cot1) and background noise. In fact, tumor DNA needs to be extracted and biotinylated, and a normal genomic DNA needs to be extracted and digoxigenin labeled, separately. After a competitive hybridization of 1 μg of DNA, tumor DNA is detected using avidin coupled to FITC (Fluorescein IsoThioCyanate), and normal DNA is detected using red-fluorescent rhodamine antidigoxigenin molecules. The sex of the patient is required for this kind of experiment in order to choose the best DNA controls to adjust X and Y for signal normalization of sex chromosomes. Depending on the ratio measurement, copy number aberrations could be identified by this method. Ratio of measurement represents: (1) normal DNA copy numbers when identical signals are quantified in green and red; (2) DNA deletions when higher signals are measures in red; and (3) DNA duplications or amplifications when signals are measured in green. CGH analysis has its limitations when it comes to balanced translocations (i.e., Ewing tumors), inversions, ring chromosomes etc. Limitations also include the sensitivity of CGH detection. Detection of small deletions is not easy and the interpretation of gains could be also difficult in specific ploidy (i.e., sarcomas, breast tumors, etc.) requiring specific bioinformatics tools.

In this context, the CGH technique was rapidly improved with the use of artificial chromosome such as BAC (bacterial artificial chromosome) (Pinkel et al. 1998), which is widely used in the Human Genome Project. Other preparations such as (Kallioniemi et al. 1994) yeast artificial chromosome (YAC), plasmid artificial chromosome (PAC), and PCR products were also used as templates for the competitive hybridization of molecules. Preparations of artificial chromosomes or PCR amplicons were controlled by sequencing before their deposition onto glass slide. Many efforts from public and private labs were engaged to set up protocols in order to improve the array designs and production of array. Principle of comparative hybridization of labeled molecules was reused to obtain the ratio of tumor DNA copy number relative to normal DNA copy number. Tumor and normal DNAs were separately fragmented using ultrasounds and coupled to specific fluorophores such as cyanine 3 or cyanine 5 (orange and red probes) before competitive hybridization.

CGH array was an evolution of CGH and facilitated high-throughput analysis of dozen of tumors, because of the use of commercial or custom-spotted glass slides (Davies et al. 2005). CGH arrays are designed with long oligonucleotides

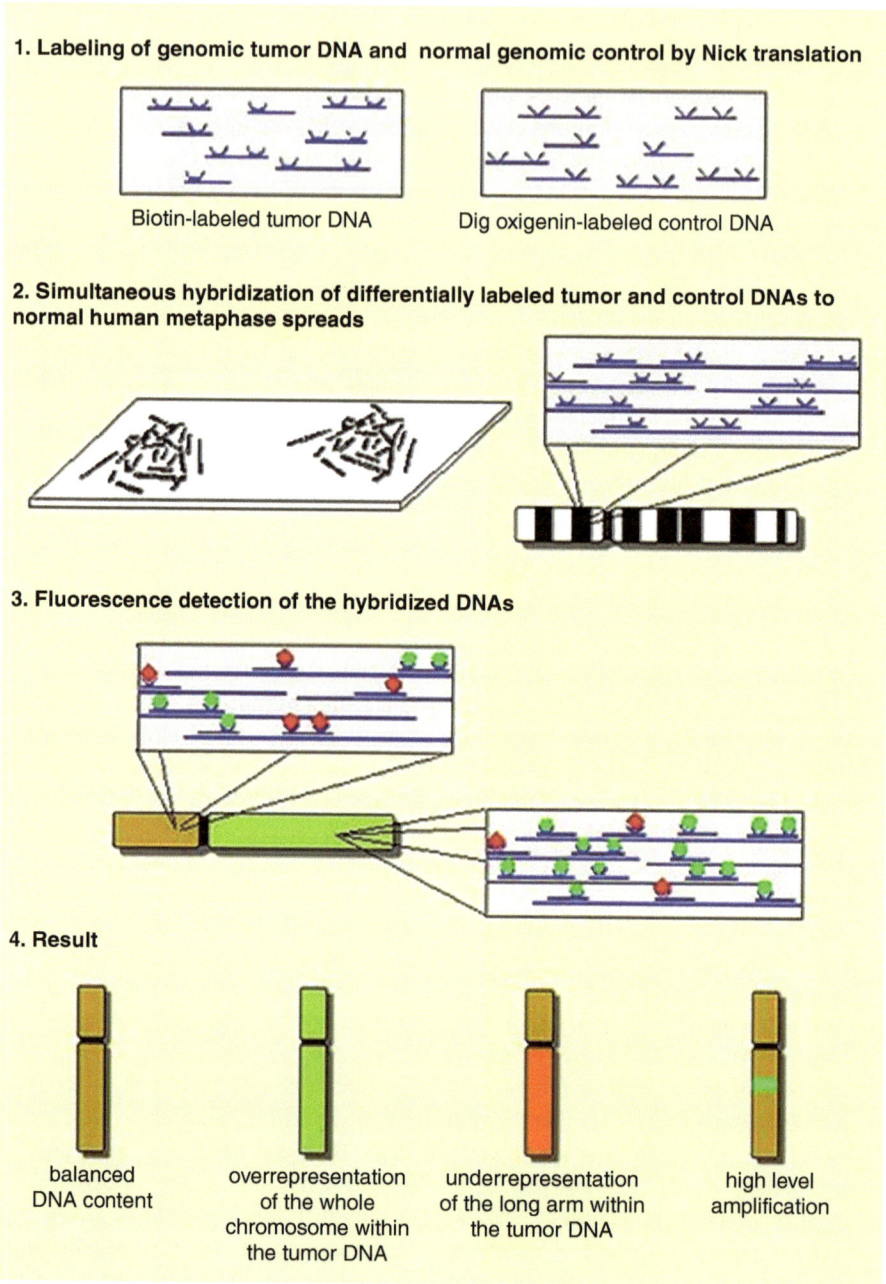

1. Labeling of genomic tumor DNA and normal genomic control by Nick translation

Biotin-labeled tumor DNA

Dig oxigenin-labeled control DNA

2. Simultaneous hybridization of differentially labeled tumor and control DNAs to normal human metaphase spreads

3. Fluorescence detection of the hybridized DNAs

4. Result

balanced DNA content

overrepresentation of the whole chromosome within the tumor DNA

underrepresentation of the long arm within the tumor DNA

high level amplification

Fig. 4.3 Principle of comparative genomic hybridization (CGH) (i.e., 60mers on Agilent technologies arrays, NimbleGen arrays) to hybridize labeled DNA. The resolution was improved to 40 kb instead of 5–10 Mb with CGH (Forozan et al. 1997), but resolution varied a lot depending on the needs. For example, Garnis et al. designed a high-content CGH arrays (Garnis et al. 2004a, b, c that quantify DNA copy number changes within a 52 Mb region of 8q21–24 to define breakpoint and limits of amplicons near *MYC* oncogene in oral dysplasia and cancer squamous cell carcinomas. Results highlighted differences in minimal altered regions, but results also confirm the need of high-content CGH array to improve accuracy on breakpoints and DNA copy number changes. The same observation was confirmed on breast tumor by Pollack et al. (2002) and on other tumor types. At this period, the Agilent Company developed genome-wide CGH arrays to analyze human genome using 60mer oligonucleotides and synthesize directly using inkjet technologies, instead of spotting BAC or PCR products.

During the development of CGH arrays, developments were also conducted on softwares to manage the intensities and algorithms to emphasize the information highlighted from complex tumors such as breast tumors.

4.4 Single Nucleotide Polymorphisms' Arrays

In parallel to CGH developments, microarrays interrogating single nucleotide polymorphism (SNP arrays) have been designed to perform high-throughput genotyping and linkage study. Affymetrix and Illumina set up two different tools to interrogate SNPs (Affymetrix mapping assays, Illumina bead array). In both tools, two alleles of selected SNP were measured using a set of probes (Affymetrix) or a single probe (Illumina) for each SNP. Fig. 4.4 extracted from T La Framboise (2009) illustrates the two different approaches that allow genotyping and DNA copy number calculations based on sequence interrogation.

Affymetrix was the first company to propose SNP arrays to characterize 12,000 SNP arrays in 1999 and to define genotypes (AA, AB, and BB), using 25mers probes. To reduce genome complexity, Affymetrix protocols were based on a first enzymatic digestion (i.e., HindIII, Xba), followed by a ligation of generic adaptors used next to PCR amplified amplicons of 100–1200 nt. Depending on the SNP assay, DNAs were next fragmented using DNAse I or using UDG/APEI complex if dUTP is incorporated in the cDNA synthesis. Fragments are next biotinylated using a specific DNA polymerase: terminal deoxynucleotidyl transferase (TdT) that binds a biotinylated nucleotide at the 3' extremity of the fragment. Those labeled molecules, corresponding to targets, are next prepared to hybridize arrays. With the improvement of technical properties of microarrays (size of features from 11 to 5 µm, scanner upgrade), the SNP array content has been amplified to 500 k. In 2007, Affymetrix has implemented non-polymorphic probes (CNV, for copy number variant) in order to improve calculation and DNA copy numbers in particular. Affymetrix SNP6.0 or CytoScan HD probes are actually interrogating ~2 M markers (900kSNP

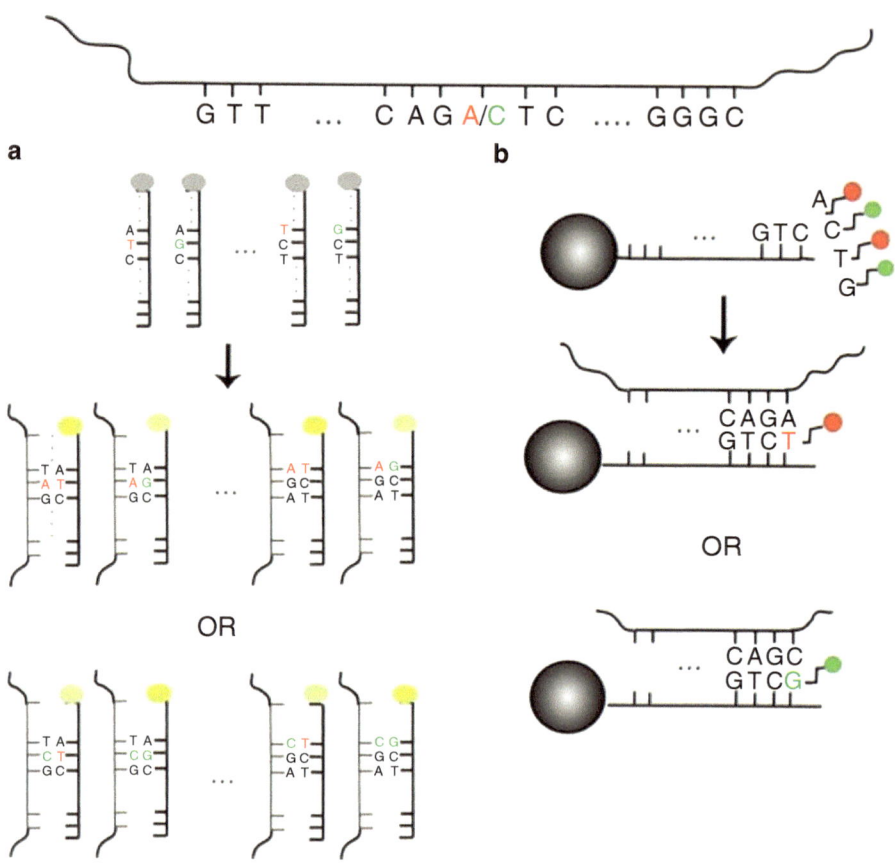

Fig. 4.4 Principle of SNP array. (**a**) Affymetrix. (**b**) Illumina (From La Framboise 2009)

and 900 k CNV in SNP6.0 array and 743 k NSP and 1.953 M CNV for CytoScan array). The improvement in terms of molecular biology consists of reduction of number of steps (one enzyme used in CytoScan instead of two for SNP6.0, 250 ng vs 500 ng as input; less PCR in CytoScan protocol). Other improvements concerned normalization steps to take into account mismatches and/or multiple probes to quantify each SNP, to assign genotypes and DNA copy numbers (i.e., BRLMM, Birdseed).

Detection of genotypes using Illumina procedures requires small amount of genomic DNA (200–400 ng) to detect specific fragments that contains SNP of interest by the mean of bead arrays (50mer probes) and dedicated protocols (GoldenGate assay, to detect between 48 and 1536 SNPs; Infinium Assay, to detect between 3072 and 1 million SNPs).

The Affymetrix tools measure in the meantime two alleles, and each sequence is interrogated onto the array, while Illumina tools are based on a competitive hybridization of a labeled nucleotide onto a bead.

Even if the first objectives to SNP arrays were to perform genotyping of SNP, their important densities were indicators of lost heterozygosity when a heterozygote state became homozygote. Other long modifications such as uniparental disomy were measureable in case of neutral DNA copy number aberrations.

The calculation of DNA copy number was another source of information when combining signal of each allele, to assign whole genome copy number and also allele specific copy number. Taking into account that the GC content infers the signal, smoothing and segmentation calculation steps were other necessary steps to use CNV probe and SNP probes to perform a whole genome copy number analysis to highlight copy number alteration, to set ploidy, for example.

4.4.1 Setup of SNP Arrays in Clinical Daily Practices

Academic genomic core facilities of cancer centers or hospitals make possible and easy the use of CGH/SNP arrays in clinical practices. For this purpose, the characterization of genomic or transcriptomic abnormalities requires a variety of competences such as platform engineers, bioinformaticians, biologists, geneticists, and medical doctors to decipher the usefulness of patients' genomic abnormalities, for personalized medicine applications as well as preclinical investigation or translational research.

Since CGH/SNP experiments require 3–5 working days, the implementation of adjusted pipelines is a must to fit the timelines of routine clinic. The setup of rapid genomic analysis requires well-identified circuits from biological resources centers (BRCs) to genomic high-throughput platforms, bioinformatics, and physicians. Preparation of genomic DNA and total RNA from fresh frozen annotated biopsies using standard procedures is one of the key steps to achieve genomic characterization. In this context, BRCs centralize nucleic acid extraction and combine histological analysis of biopsies. Based on H&E staining of a thin frozen tissue section, the tumor cell percentage is estimated by pathologists. In most of array-based approaches, the threshold of the tumor cell percentage is fixed to 30 or 50 % corresponding to the limit of detection of abnormalities (losses and gains) within tumor cells. This parameter is important and can reject sample because of a lack of tumor cells in samples. In the Safir01 trial (André et al. 2014), 22.5 % (91/403) of biopsies were excluded due to a lack of tumor cells. Another important point is the amount of genomic DNA available from biopsy. As most of SNP array requires 250–500 ng of genomic DNA, fine needle aspiration or small biopsies could lead to low yield of extraction. In this context, whole genome amplification (WGA) protocol may overcome to low amount of DNA used for genomic analysis. This process is based on a modified phi29 enzymes that amplify genomic DNA (gDNA). WGA requires at least 10–30 ng of DNA to generate micrograms of DNA (Fig. 4.5). This pre-processing of gDNA can also generate artifact of measurements (Fig 4.6a) on repetitive sequences, telomeres, etc. In the Safir01 trial, whole genome amplification was

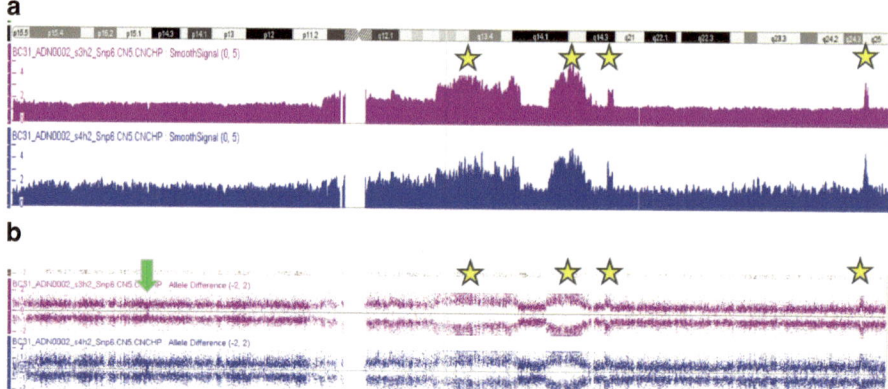

Fig. 4.5 Example of breast tumor analyzed on SNP6.0 Affymetrix arrays (zoomed on chr11). Purple tracks correspond to experiment started with 500 ng of gDNA, and blue tracks correspond to experiment started with preamplified DNA using WGA process (same sample). (**a**) The smooth signal tracks correspond to copy numbers, and gains labeled with yellow stars are found in both conditions. Smooth signal is varying a little bit more in the blue track corresponding to the preamplified DNA. (**b**) Allele differences are similar in both conditions: LOH and gains (*yellow stars*) are found in both cases. A small deletion (*green arrow*) is found in both samples (unamplified and preamplified DNA°)

applied when few nanograms of DNA were available. Results were successfully analyzed on SNP array for 30 % of samples, and other cases failed because results did not allow recognition of clear DNA copy numbers changes.

Another aspect of the implementation of SNP arrays in routine clinical practice concerns the validation of data generated. As SNP arrays were designed for genotyping analysis of normal DNA, analysis of tumors makes invalid default manufacturer quality criteria. In practice and concerning genomic tumor profiling, SNP call rates could be below than expected due to losses, allelic models (AA, AB, BB), and their representation need to be adjusted because of aberrant ploidy (Affymetrix parameters such as contrast QC and MAPD are often out of specification when complex tumors samples are analyzed). In this context, having a normal DNA analyzed in parallel of tumor samples is important to check the quality of each experiment. The absence of genomic abnormalities is necessary to validate the absence of any tumor DNA contamination. Next, the analysis of copy number states and allelic imbalance (nor LOH) is important to conclude on genome abnormalities.

4.5   New Arrays Based on Molecular Inversion Probes

Frozen tissues or living cells generate good quality CGH and SNP arrays because in most of cases, the integrity of gDNA is preserved. Nevertheless, analysis of degraded DNA from formalin-fixed, paraffin-embedded (FFPE) tissues is much

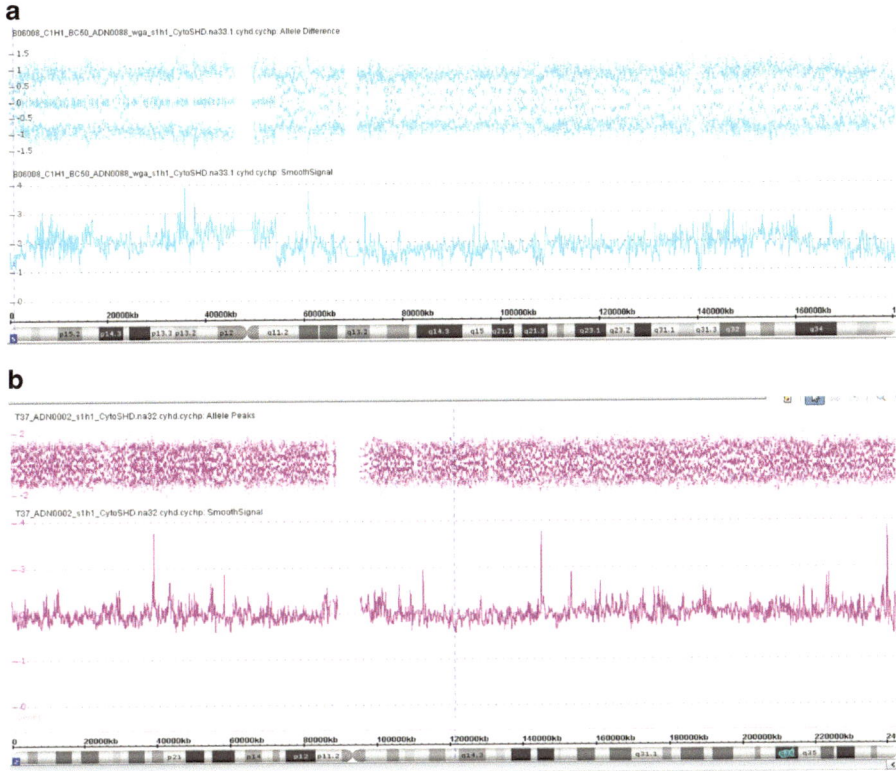

Fig. 4.6 Example of poor-quality data. (**a**) A tumor DNA was purified from a FFPE tumor, pre-amplified using a WGA, and analyzed on SNP array. The smooth copy number and allelic difference on chromosome 5 are noisy: A lot of peaks are detected on the smooth signal track, and allele difference may reflect genomic abnormalities and cellular heterogeneity. Altogether, those results cannot be interpreted. (**b**) A tumor DNA was purified from a FFPE tumor and analyzed on SNP6 array (chr2). The smooth copy number and allelic difference on chromosome 2 are noisy: A lot of pictures are detected on the smooth signal track, and allele differences are noisy too. Those data were not useful

more difficult due the fixative solution and deparaffinization steps that alter genome (size fragmentation; genome hydrolysis, i.e., *depurination*; *etc*.). In this context (Fig. 4.6b), DNA copy number determination is not possible due to artifacts of measurement and presence of abnormal copy number peaks. The analysis performed at the allelic level is also impossible and allelic status cannot be determined. To overcome poor-quality DNA, Wang et al. in 2012 proposed another strategy based on molecular inversion probes (MIP) to detect SNP, copy numbers, and LOH. The MIP protocol was proposed in 1994 by Nilsson et al. (1994) to detect DNA and implemented by Hardenbol et al. (2003) to amplify circularized probes, in order to perform multiplexed genotyping as proposed by Wang Y et al. (2012) (Fig. 4.7a).

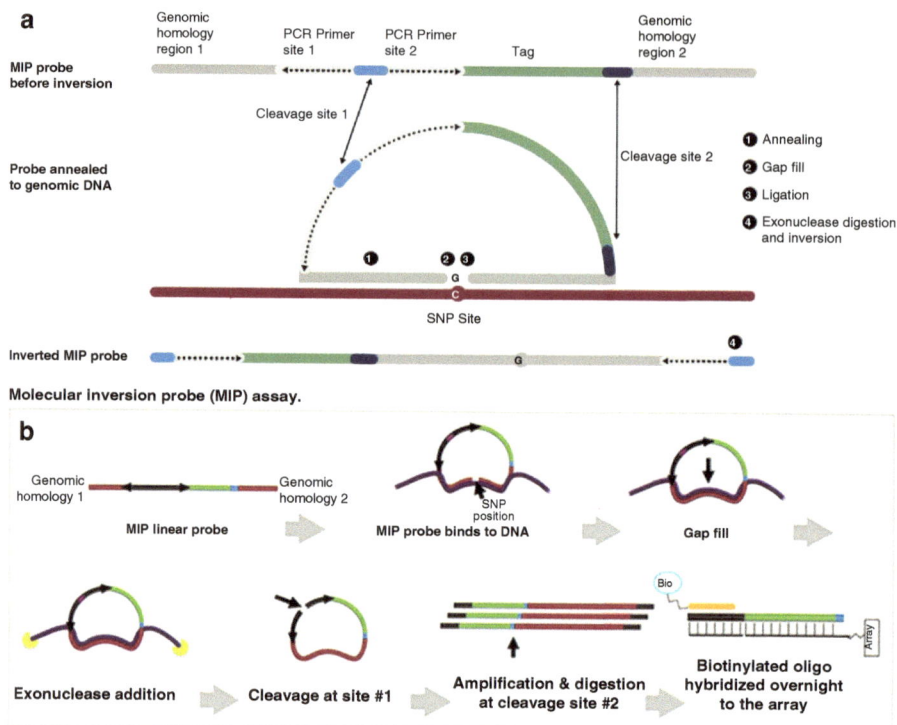

Fig. 4.7 Principle of molecular inversion probe: (**a**) description of the MIP principle (From Wang et al. 2012). (**b**) Description of the MIP Affymetrix assay used to hybridize OncoScan arrays

The Affymetrix OncoScan assay (Fig. 4.7b) used the molecular inversion probe technology which interrogated 220.000 regions among the genome, with a 50–100 kb copy number resolution in 900 oncogenes and 300 kb genome-wide copy number resolution outside oncogenes. Briefly, MIP probes are annealed to 30–80 ng gDNA derived from fixed tissues. Probes are designed with a gap (of a single nucleotide) delimited by the hybridized ends of the probes (~40 nt each) that remains over the target region. Each DNA is split in two wells, and the reaction to fill the gap (at the SNP position) is processed by adding dATP/dTTP to one well and dCTP/dGTP to another well. Uncircularized MIP probes are digested by an exonuclease, in order to keep only MIP probes that have been gap filled by the A/T or G/C nucleotides. The circular MIP probes are then linearized using a cleavage enzyme and amplified by PCR. 125pb PCR amplicons are generated and controlled by electrophoresis before a second PCR, followed by a HAEIII enzyme digestion, to generate small fragments that will be hybridized on OncoScan arrays. This approach is suitable to analyze fragmented DNA (Fig. 4.8a) extracted from FFPE samples, from cytological specimen, and also from circulating DNA (Fig. 4.8b). Concerning FFPE samples, DNA can be extracted using dedicated protocol (i.e., QIAamp DNA FFPE Tissue Kit) from FFPE sections (10–50 μm thick), laser microdissection of large

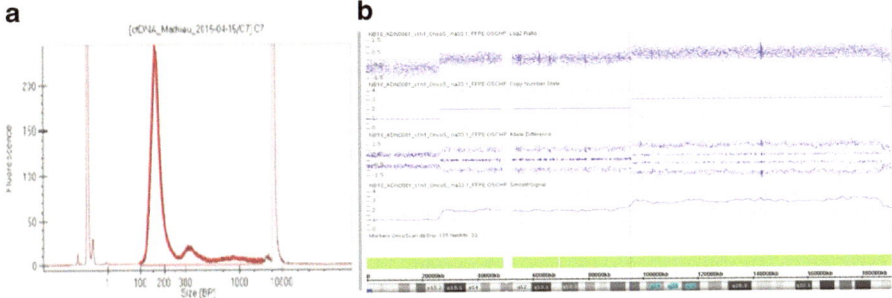

Fig. 4.8 Analysis of a ctDNA extracted from plasma hybridized on MIP array. (**a**) Circulating DNA extracted from plasma was controlled on LabChip, Bioanalyzer. (**b**) 80 ng of ctDNA was used to hybridize Affymetrix OncoScan array. Chromosome 4 profile shows clear copy of number alterations (loss and gains). Allele differences are also very clear for each copy number state (1, 2, and 3 copies, corresponding to A or B; AA, AB, and BB; and AAA, AAB, ABB, BBB states)

area from a stained FFPE section. DNA can also be extracted from scrapped cells on stained FFPE sections or stained cytological specimen.

4.6 Conclusion and Challenges

The use of microarrays in routine clinical practices is now admitted for patient management and precision medicine to identify gains (*MYCN*) and losses (*PTEN*) of specific genes related to "targeted" pathways.

Furthermore, the global analysis of copy number abnormalities was helpful to highlight genomic instability. For example, Dr. Popova T and Dr. MH Stern used copy numbers, LOHs through the GAP algorithm to determine the ploidy and to characterize genomic abnormalities according to the nearest observed ploidy (adjusted gains and losses). This first step analysis allows authors to define a signature related to large-scale genomic instability (Popova et al. 2009). This signature was evaluated in series of breast cancers and breast cancer cell lines. Number of chromosomal breaks between adjacent regions of several sizes was monitored, and large-scale state transition (LST) was defined in at least 10 Mb for near diploid and near tetraploid breast carcinomas. High score of LST (at 10 Mb) predicted *BRCA1/2* inactivation and may reflect a rapid and cost-effective tool, relative to genetic testing that aims to measure inactivation of BRCA genes at several levels (genetic or epigenetic inactivation).

Even if most of the array content is fixed to known events compared to genome-wide sequencing approaches and even if results correspond or not to attempted results (lack of genomic alterations, genome instability), their use in daily routine is robust with the help of controls and standard samples and requires know-how and knowledge of tumor genomic characterization.

The SNP arrays are actually a complementary tool to exome/targeted sequencing to achieve precise and cost-effective analysis, in a time-lapse compatibility to clinical daily practices. The amount of required material is still a point of improvement to detect rare event from any sources of specimen (serum, urines, and other fluids). The type of alterations detected by SNP arrays needs also to be implemented to known event (indels, translocation) and needs also to be customized upon request in order to quantify specific sequences as the MIP approach should propose; otherwise, direct molecules sequencing and quantification will be applied.

In order to reconstruct and understand tumor complexity, genomic data and clinical and biological annotation needed to be collected and discussed with a board of biologists, bioinformaticians, and clinicians. Improvement in tumor complexity understanding should facilitate the identification of driver genes and passenger genes for personalized medicine.

Acknowledgments Thanks to Cécile Reyes, Emilie Henry, and Audrey Rapinat for providing illustrations of samples they analyzed for the genomic core facility. Thanks to Dr. Gudrun Schleiermacher, MD PhD, and Chicard Mathieu for their collaboration on ctDNA.

References

André F, Bachelot T, Commo F et al (2014) Comparative genomic hybridisation array and DNA sequencing to direct treatment of metastatic breast cancer: a multicentre, prospective trial (SAFIR01/UNICANCER). Lancet Oncol 15(3):267–274. doi:10.1016/S1470-2045(13)70611-9. Epub 2014 Feb 7

Bickmore WA (2001) Karyotype analysis and chromosome banding. Nature. doi:10.1038/npg. els.0001160

Davies JJ, Wilson IM, Lam WL (2005) Array CGH technologies and their applications to cancer genomes. Chromosome Res 13(3):237–248

Ferguson-Smith MA (2008) Cytogenetics and the evolution of medical genetics. Genet Med 10:553–559, doi:10.1097

Forozan F, Karhu R, Kononen J et al (1997) Genome screening by comparative genomic hybridization. Trends Genet 13:405–409

Gad S, Aurias A, Puget N et al (2001) Color bar coding the *BRCA1* gene on combed DNA: a useful strategy for detecting large gene rearrangements. Genes Chromosomes Cancer 31(1):75–84

Gad S, Klinger M, Caux-Moncoutier V et al (2002) Bar code screening on combed DNA for large rearrangements of the *BRCA1* and BRCA2 genes in French breast cancer families. J Med Genet 39(11):817–821

Gall JG, Pardue ML (1969) Formation and detection of RNA-DNA hybrid molecules in cytological preparations. Proc Natl Acad Sci U S A A63(2):378–383

Garnis C, Coe BP, Ishkanian A et al (2004a) Novel regions of amplification on 8q distinct from the *MYC* locus and frequently altered in oral dysplasia and cancer. Genes Chromosomes Cancer 39:93–98

Garnis C, Coe BP, Zhang L et al (2004b) Overexpression of LRP12, a gene contained within an 8q22 amplicon identified by high-resolution array CGH analysis of oral squamous cell carcinomas. Oncogene 23:2582–2586

Garnis C, MacAulay C, Lam S et al (2004c) Genetic alteration on 8q distinct from *MYC* in bronchial carcinoma in situ lesions. Lung Cancer 44:403–404

Hardenbol P, Banér J, Jain M et al (2003) Multiplexed genotyping with sequence-tagged molecular inversion probes. Nat Biotechnol 21(6):673–678, Epub 2003 May 5

Harper PS (2006) The discovery of the human chromosome number in Lund, 1955–1956. Hum Genet 119(1–2):226–232

International HapMap Consortium (2003) The international HapMap project. Nature 426(6968):789–796

John HA, Birnstiel ML, Jones KW (1969) RNA-DNA hybrids at the cytological level. Nature 223(5206):582–587

Kallioniemi A, Kallioniemi OP, Sudar D et al (1992) Comparative genomic hybridization for molecular cytogenetic analysis of solid tumors. Science 258(5083):818–821

Kallioniemi OP, Kallioniemi A, Piper J et al (1994) Optimizing comparative genomic hybridization for analysis of DNA sequence copy number changes in solid tumors. Genes Chromosomes Cancer 10:231–243

La Framboise T (2009) Single nucleotide polymorphism arrays: a decade of biological, computational and technological advances. Nucleic Acids Res 37(13):4181–4193. doi:10.1093/nar/gkp552. Epub 2009 Jul 1

Langer-Safer PR, Levine M, Ward DC (1982) Immunological method for mapping genes on Drosophila polytene chromosomes. Proc Natl Acad Sci U S A 79(14):4381–4385

Nilsson M, Malmgren H, Samiotaki M et al (1994) Padlock probes: circularizing oligonucleotides for localized DNA detection. Science 265(5181):2085–2088. doi:10.1126/science.7522346

Pinkel D, Segraves R, Sudar D et al (1998) High resolution analysis of DNA copy number variation using comparative genomic hybridization to microarrays. Nat Genet 20:207–211

Pollack JR, Sorlie T, Perou CM et al (2002) Microarray analysis reveals a major direct role of DNA copy number alteration in the transcriptional program of human breast tumors. Proc Natl Acad Sci U S A 99:12963–12968

Popova T, Manié E, Stoppa-Lyonnet D et al (2009) Genome Alteration Print (GAP): a tool to visualize and mine complex cancer genomic profiles obtained by SNP arrays. Genome Biol 10(11):R128. doi:10.1186/gb-2009-10-11-r128. Epub 2009 Nov 11

Ried T, Schröck E, Ning Y et al (1998) Chromosome painting: a useful art. Hum Mol Genet 7(10):1619–1626

Singer MF (1982) SINEs and LINEs: highly repeated short and long interspersed sequences in mammalian genomes. Cell 28(3):433–434

Volpi EV, Bridger JM (2008) FISH glossary: an overview of the fluorescence in situ hybridization technique. Biotechniques 45:385–409

Wang Y, Cottman M, Schiffman JD (2012) Molecular inversion probes: a novel microarray technology and its application in cancer research. Cancer Genet 205(7–8):341–355. doi:10.1016/j.cancergen.2012.06.005

Waye JS, Willard HF (1986) Structure, organization, and sequence of alpha satellite DNA from human chromosome 17: evidence for evolution by unequal crossing-over and an ancestral pentamer repeat shared with the human X chromosome. Mol Cell Biol 6(9):3156–3165

Weiner AM (2002) SINEs and LINEs: the art of biting the hand that feeds you. Curr Opin Cell Biol 14(3):343–350

Weiss M, Hermsen M, Meijer G et al (1999) Comparative genomic hybridization. Mol Pathol 52:243–251

Chapter 5
High-Throughput Technologies: DNA and RNA Sequencing Strategies and Potential

Thomas Rio Frio

5.1 The Next-Generation Sequencing and Its Impact on Genomics and Clinical Genetic Testing

5.1.1 Early DNA Sequencing

Nucleic acid sequencing is a key tool for scientific research and clinical diagnosis to understand and decipher the code to all biological life on earth as well as to understand and treat genetic diseases. DNA and RNA are made up of four chemical bases or nucleotides arranged in different ways to constitute the genes. Sequencing is the process to determine the order of these nucleotides in one or more targeted regions. Several sequencing methods were developed in the 1970s, and the approach developed by Frederick Sanger in 1977, rewarded by a Noble Prize in chemistry in 1980, revolutionized the field of genomics (Sanger et al. 1977). The method called chain-termination method or dideoxynucleotide sequencing consists in the polymerization of DNA fragments complementary to a DNA template, using a mix of deoxynucleotide triphosphate (dNTP), the building blocks for DNA, and fluorescent dideoxynucleotide triphosphate (ddNTP). These ddNTPs or terminators emit each light at different wavelengths depending on their nature (ddATP, ddTTP, ddCTP, ddGTP) and prevent the addition of other dNTPs. The synthesis of complementary DNA strand stops when a ddNTP is randomly incorporated, leading to as many different fragments ending each with a fluorescent ddNTPs as the length of the DNA fragment to sequence. Products from this sequencing reaction are then migrated by electrophoresis in capillaries to separate fragments based on their size,

T. Rio Frio, PhD
Genoma SA, NGS Platform, Geneva, Switzerland
e-mail: thomas.rio-frio@genoma.com

© Springer International Publishing Switzerland 2015
C. Le Tourneau, M. Kamal (eds.), *Pan-cancer Integrative Molecular Portrait*
Towards a New Paradigm in Precision Medicine,
DOI 10.1007/978-3-319-22189-2_5

47

and a laser reads the ending fluorescent ddNTP. Successive fluorescent signals allow reconstituting the sequence of the fragment analyzed. DNA fragments of maximum 1–1.2 kb can be accurately sequenced. Different versions of Sanger-based sequencer were released, from one capillary to 96 capillaries. The configuration with the highest throughput per instrument allows 96 samples to be run simultaneously with 24–36 runs per day, which represents a throughput of 1–2 million bases per day. The Sanger-based sequencing method has been extensively used in research and for genetic testing since its development and made possible one of the major scientific achievements, the sequencing of the human genome.

5.1.2   The Human Genome Project

The Human Genome Project (HGP) was a large international collaborative research project started in 1990 and that lasted for 13 years. It involved six countries (France, Germany, Japan, China, UK, and USA) and cost $2.7 billion (https://www.genome. gov/10001772). The goal of this project was to decode the human genome and to create a vast resource of detailed scientific information about the structural organization and function of human DNA. Steps of the project consisted first in the generation of the physical and genetic maps of the human genome, second, in the determination of the complete sequence of the human genome, and third in the identification and mapping of genes. The sequencing of model organisms such as *M. Musculus*, *E. coli*, and *D. melanogaster* as well as conducting functional studies to develop genomic-scale technologies were also part of the project. The first draft of the human genome was published in Nature in 2001 (International Human Genome Sequencing Consortium 2001), and the project was declared officially complete in April 2003 with 99 % of gene-containing part of human sequence finished with 99.99 % accuracy (International Human Genome Sequencing Consortium 2004). The HGP revealed that the size of the genome is 3 billion bases and that it contains around 20,500 genes, but this number may still slightly fluctuate. The human reference genome is freely and publicly available for scientific purposes, and further analyses are still ongoing to treat few refractory problems, such as large repetitive DNA regions.

   To achieve this project that required the sequencing of long DNA sections, a new approach using the Sanger-based sequencing method, called hierarchical shotgun sequencing, was developed. Genomic DNA was enzymatically or mechanically broken into 100–200 kilobase pieces and cloned into bacterial hosts using vectors. Clones that reconstituted the human genome with the minimum tiling path were selected, sheared in smaller fragments, and sequenced by Sanger-based method. The complete sequence of the human genome was then possible to reassemble based on partial overlap of generated sequences using specific bioinformatics tools (Waterston et al. 2002).

   This major scientific achievement marked the beginning of the post-genomic area. Since the completion of the first human genome and with the availability of a reference sequence, scientific research aims now to annotate and functionally characterize genes; understand gene-gene interactions, regulation of gene expression, and protein-protein interactions; and apply this knowledge to better understand life and to predict, prevent, and cure diseases. Demand for faster and cheaper sequencing methods has since dramatically increased, and powerful genomic tools became a mandatory condition to achieve these goals. Several academic laboratories as well as biotechnology companies worked on high-throughput sequencing methods based on the shotgun approach and gave rise to next-generation sequencing technology.

5.1.3   The Next-Generation Sequencing Revolution

Similarly to Sanger-based sequencing method, next-generation sequencing (NGS) is the result of multiple developments and optimization of existing method before the launch of the first next-generation DNA sequencer by 454 Life Sciences in 2005 (Margulies et al 2005). The core philosophy behind all NGS methods developed so far is the simultaneous sequencing of million to billions of short DNA molecules in a same reaction that dramatically increases the throughput and reduces cost compared to Sanger-based method. The actual most powerful NGS system, the HiSeq X Ten System from Illumina, can produce up to 6 billion of sequences per 3-day runs and per instrument. It represents 1,000 times the throughput of the most powerful configuration of an instrument running Sanger-based sequencing method. From 2001 to 2007, along with the optimization of Sanger-based associated technology, the cost per megabase (1,000,000 DNA bases) of sequence went from $10 K down to $600 (94 % reduction) (https://www.genome.gov/sequencingcosts/). This cost dropped dramatically from $600 in 2007 to $0.1 (99.98 % reduction) within the next 4 years along with the launch of NGS sequencers and their fast evolution. The sequencing of a whole human genome can now be achieved in 1 day with one sequencer and costs $1,000, whereas it took 13 years for an international collaboration and $2.7B to sequence the first human genome. This huge decrease of sequencing costs leads to an extraordinary boost of scientific research and exponential growth of sequencing data produced. Contrary to Sanger-based sequencing for which the sequencing signal is derived from all molecules in the reaction, NGS technology sequences every DNA fragment enriched by sample preparation individually. A mixture of DNA molecules derived from different genomic targets can be then sequenced in a same sequencing run. Furthermore, a molecular barcode is usually added in all fragments derived from each DNA sample during preparation of sequencing templates. Thus, several genomic targets from several individuals can be sequenced simultaneously. Bioinformatic analysis of sequenced data attributes sequencing reads to every sample based on the analysis of the molecular barcode and to the region on the reference genome to find from which sequence it derived. This characteristic of NGS allows the quantification of variants detected in sequences and not only their detection as with Sanger-based method. Detection of low-level mutations, below 10 %, which is the common admitted detection limit of Sanger sequencing, is therefore possible with NGS that actually has depending on the sequencer a detection limit of 0.5–1 %. Fine genetic analysis of collected tumoral tissues that are usually contaminated with healthy surrounding tissue is possible.

5.1.4   The Impact of Next-Generation Sequencing

5.1.4.1   Scientific Research

Surfing on the success of the Human Genome Project, first NGS sequencers were designed primarily to scientific research and not intended to a clinical use. NGS has been extensively used for *de novo* sequencing of a broad range of biological organisms, from microbial to human (animals, plants, bacteria, yeasts, etc.), and provides insights into genome, epigenome, and transcriptome that allows the understanding of these organisms. Because of mild high throughput, mostly bacteria and yeast genomes that are relatively small (<1–15 Mb) and their transcriptomes were studied (Farrer et al. 2009). In microbiology, NGS has facilitated the study of the correlation between genotype and phenotype in these widely used genetic models that contribute significantly to the understanding of human genome and genetic diseases. NGS also helps to optimize food safety and process and health management (accurate identification of bacterial infection, helps to manage epidemic diseases). Along with the increase of sequencing throughput and bioinformatics development, larger genomes such as human and mouse genomes (~3.10^9 base pairs both) have been extensively sequenced (1000 Genomes Project Consortium et al. 2010) to improve the reference genome sequence, to study genetic diseases, and to decipher the function of genes, their organization, their regulation, and their evolution. For example, targeted sequencing of exome, the complete coding part of the genome, revealed causal genetic mutations for rare congenital syndromes, intellectual disability, autism, and schizophrenia (Rabbani et al. 2012). NGS has been extensively used in cancer research in the past few years to detect a number of novel cancer-related genes with the sequencing of large sample cohorts through international collaborations. To achieve a high-resolution view of cancer genomes, several NGS-based methods were developed (whole genome sequencing, exome sequencing, transcriptome sequencing, ChIP-seq, etc.),and the combination of these technologies allowed the detection of novel genetic alterations, point mutations, small insertions or deletions, copy number alterations, and structural variations that contribute to oncogenesis, tumor development, and metastasis (Shyr and Liu 2013). NGS was also able to get insight in the tumor genomic intra-heterogeneity through its high detection and quantification resolution. More complex and larger genomes such as in plants (10^9–10^{11} base pairs) often contain large portions of repetitive sequences and transposable elements. Furthermore, polyploidy is common in these organisms, adding another layer of complexity in the study of such genomes. The use of NGS made possible the sequencing of these genomes with multiple genomes released since 2007 (rice, maize, banana, cacao, etc.). Variants influencing significantly valuable phenotypic traits have been identified, and the agriculture benefits from these findings (Berkman et al. 2012). In archeology and paleontology, NGS has been successfully used for the sequencing of ancient DNA to reconstruct patterns of evolution and to study population genetics and paleontological changes. For example, the generation of high-quality genomes of a Neanderthal individual and other archaic hominins was performed with the use of NGS and helps to clarify temporal and spatial human evolution (Sánchez-Quinto and Lalueza-Fox 2015). NGS has had also a big impact on metagenomics, which is the study of the total genomic content of a microbial community, for example, in the human gut. The high-throughput capability, relatively low cost, and depth of next-generation sequencing make such study easier by avoiding the need to isolate populations who introduced experimental biased. Through NGS approaches, new species were detected and microbial diversity as well as relative abundance could be assessed with a high resolution that has contributed to the understanding of species and functions present in a microbial community (Thomas et al. 2012). A lot of various scientific research fields have benefited from this powerful genomic tool, and further applications are continuously developed to enlarge the spectrum of NGS applications in research.

5.1.4.2 Clinical Genetic Testing

In the years 2000, Sanger-based sequencing was the gold standard for clinical genetic testing because of its high robustness proven through decades of results in research and clinical genetic testing, its ease of use, and ease of analysis. The complexity to run NGS sequencers, the significant failure rate, mild sequencing quality (reduced length of sequencing reads, significant error rate), as well as few available bioinformatics tools prevented the setup of these instruments for clinical diagnosis. The throughput was also too high to simply translate clinical genetic tests performed on Sanger-based sequencers as this time leading to increase costs for similar test. Bioinformatics analysis of generated sequence data was in its early days; no robust ready-to-use and user-friendly solution was available to ensure highest specificity and sensitivity of genetic tests. As for any technological revolution, NGS sequencers evolved quickly with chemistry, workflow, and bioinformatics, with significant optimizations released on a yearly basis. Quality of generated data dramatically improved, opening the possibility of using NGS sequencers in a clinical setting. In parallel to the development of sequencers with higher throughput dedicated to scientific research, sequencing manufacturer developed clinically oriented sequencers with the goal to conquer the highly profitable clinical market. These sequencers were designed as benchtop sequencers. They are relatively small and user-friendly equipment running with reduced manual operations, and they require little maintenance. The throughput is also reduced to fit with genetic testing requirement, the main goal being not the sequencing of genomes but to sequences selected targets with clinical interest. In the meantime, bioinformatics solutions improved significantly and were proven to be robust for the detection of variants. In 2013 the US Food and Drug Administration authorized broad clinical use of the MiSeqDx DNA sequencing system from Illumina, the first NGS sequencer to be certified for *in vitro diagnostic* use (http://www.fda.gov/NewsEvents/Newsroom/PressAnnouncements/ucm375742.htm). Later, in 2014, the FDA cleared the Ion Torrent PGM as a medical device (http://news.thermofisher.com/press-release/life-technologies/thermo-fisher-scientific-announces-listing-ion-pgm-dx-system-us-fda-). However, certifications remain limited regarding the versatility of NGS sequencers since only the sequencing of cystic fibrosis-associated gene *CFTR* on the MiSeq is certified and only few run configurations and throughputs are certified. Consequently, many laboratories and biotechnology companies across the world have developed their own sequencing NGS-based tests such as gene sequencing panels and run those in clinical routine despite a lack of certification of NGS processes.

Several companies such as Life Technologies, Illumina, Agilent, and Roche developed reliable and robust solutions to enrich genomic and RNA targets. They and others propose ready-to-use gene enrichment panels with clinical interest or user-friendly solutions to design customized gene panels. For example, the enrichment of human exome that represents the coding part of the genome is used both in research and clinics to search for unsuspected molecular abnormalities in case of genetic disease, and the sequencing of *CFTR* gene is performed for the detection of cystic fibrosis. With these targeted sequencing solutions, laboratories could move from the analysis of a portion of a gene to the screening of a full gene and even more to tens of genes at the same time allowing a most comprehensive clinical screening which was restricted because of cost, time, and hard setup. Sanger-based method is still used but mostly to confirm variants detected by NGS that could be challenging for some NGS sequencers, for example, an insertion/deletion in long homopolymer stretches. Many clinical genetic centers have already reconfigured their diagnostic processes and adopted NGS as the preferred technology for the diagnosis of diseases (genome, exome, or targeted sequencing). For example, Children Hospital of Philadelphia started to run clinical exomes on children with rare conditions, unexplained despite extensive investigations (http://pediseq.research.chop.edu/). Exome has been extensively used in research, and actual knowledge makes it valuable for the assessment of genetic diseases in newborns. This type of study would permit the estimation of the benefit of exome sequencing compared to conventional medical approach as well as its economical impact.

Actually, the main clinical NGS-based application is noninvasive prenatal testing (NIPT) with an estimated one million of samples processed in the world in 2014 and with an expected market value of $3.62 billion in 2019 (Dondorp et al. 2015). In the 1990s, cell-free DNA derived from placental cells has been found to circulate in the maternal blood during pregnancy (Lo et al. 1997). The fetal DNA represents at least 4 % of total cell-free DNA at 10th week of pregnancy subsequently increases along with maternal age and totally disappears in few hours after delivery (Wang et al. 2013; Bianchi et al. 2012, 2014). The tri-test currently performed during the first trimester of pregnancy is based on biochemical analysis and measurement of nuchal translucency. It gives a high portion of false positives and false negatives. False-positive cases are referred to unnecessary amniocentesis with a risk of miscarriage of 1 %, and false-negative cases prevent from the evaluation of a possible termination of pregnancy. With the high throughput and quantitative property of NGS sequencers, sequencing circulating cell-free DNA extracted from maternal blood plasma and detecting the presence of chromosomal numerical abnormalities with a sensitivity and specificity close to 100 % are possible. NIPT is actually able to call trisomies of chromosomes 13, 18, and 21 as well as sex chromosome aneuploidies. It is also able to determine the sex of the fetus with accuracy close to 100 % (Devers et al. 2013). Briefly, circulating cell-free DNA (mother + fetus) is sequenced and reads counted on each chromosome. After normalization on chromosome length and GC content, a departure from expected quantity of reads corresponding to half of the fetal fraction indicates an aneuploidy of the fetus. NIPT remains informative since the fetal DNA analyzed is derived from the placenta and not from the fetus. Despite the high sensitivity and specificity of NIPT, some false-positive cases happen mostly because of confined placental mosaicism or vanishing twin. An amniocentesis is recommended in case of a positive result, but the low rate of false negative and false positive compared to conventional tri-test makes NIPT a real improvement for prenatal screening. Most recent version of NIPT can detect microdeletions with a resolution down to 5 Mb that is at least equivalent if not better than amniocentesis. However, NIPT as well as other genetic test currently performed using NGS are considered as laboratory developed tests which neither need to be regulated nor certified by FDA in the USA. Major sequencing players have invested this business such as Verinata (Illumina), BGI, Ariosa (Roche), as well as new biotechnology companies such as Genoma and Premaitha. The fast implementation of NIPT in the clinical practice worldwide demonstrates that NGS has started to revolutionize clinical genetic diagnosis. Many other NGS clinical applications are actually evaluated to determine their contribution to diagnosis and treatment selection.

In clinical oncology, whole genome sequencing is considered as the unbiased gold standard to give a high-resolution view of alterations and structure of the genome (Bennett et al. 2014; Bianchi et al. 2014). Because of the size of the human genome and the associated cost, a comprehensive study of the heterogeneity of analyzed tumor remains difficult to perform routinely. Actually, analysis is restricted to the sequencing of some genetic regions or genes in which alterations are known to promote cancer progression. For example, *BRCA1* and *BRCA2*, two genes strongly implicated in hereditary breast and ovarian cancers, are screened in some laboratories only for some well-documented mutations, and some laboratories analyze the complete coding sequence of these genes. A nonnegligible portion of hereditary breast and ovarian cancers are not linked to these two genes, and the screening of other candidate genes such as *TP53, PALB2, CHEK2,* etc., allows to perform an all-in-one analysis of patients and to avoid a time-consuming iterative strategy gene after gene. For example, Myriad Genetics, the world leader in *BRCA1* and *BRCA2* analysis, performed their sequencing using Sanger-based method. Myriad shifted this test to NGS and proposed now the analysis of several genes by NGS to evaluate predisposition of some other hereditary cancers (colorectal, melanoma, etc.). With the $1,000 human genome, systematic sequencing of the tumoral genome and normal tissue as reference appears to be the next standard medical practice. Such approach would allow the personalization of treatment based on genomic alterations detected avoiding unnecessary and painful inefficient treatments. Unfortunately, the clinical significance of variants detected in whole genome studies remains actually challenging. Extensive sequencing of cohorts of individuals (1000 genome project, 100,000 UK genomes project, etc.), several types of tumors (The Cancer Genome Atlas) are ongoing and would help to refine analysis in a close future and to give better interpretation of sequencing data. Sequencing of circulating cell-free DNA seems a promising approach to indirectly track tumor progression (Lianos et al. 2015). It has been recently shown that DNA from certain types and stages of tumors circulates in the blood of the patient. Through the analysis of the circulating cell-free DNA by NGS, studies have shown that it was possible to detect mutations previously identified in the tumor through a simple liquid biopsy (Lebofsky et al. 2015). It is still too early to use this technique to detect cancer, but this strategy would be of use to monitor tumor treatment by following the evolution of the presence of the mutation in circulating cell-free DNA of patients.

Primarily dedicated to research, NGS has started to unravel its huge potential for clinical applications. Nevertheless, despite its major role in major scientific achievements, NGS is still in development. Some technological issues remain to be fixed to get sequencing tool that fulfills all quality requirements for high-throughput clinical genetic testing. Furthermore, crucial points need to be addressed regarding the use of NGS in clinical diagnostic, incidental findings in case of exome or genome sequencing, genetic profiling for health insurance, and eugenics. It is actually possible to sequence the whole genome of a preimplantation embryo and to select embryos based on nonmedical traits, such as stature, memory, hair and eye color, or athletic ability. NGS is a powerful genomic tool for genomics that has revolutionized scientific research, but strong regulation of its use in clinical settings is required.

5.2   The Next-Generation Sequencers

Laboratory workflow is similar for all actual NGS platforms from the second generation of sequencers. It is divided in 3 phases: (1) preparation of sequencing libraries starting from purified DNA or RNA, (2) library immobilization and clonal amplification, and (3) sequencing. NGS sequencers are able to reconstitute the sequence of several billions of DNA fragments simultaneously but have some restrictions regarding the length of sequenced DNA fragments and the size of sequencing reads. Indeed, DNA fragments cannot exceed 300–500 bp on average and depending on the instrument. The length of sequencing reads is usually restricted to 100–250 nucleotides depending on the sequencing chemistry used and sequencing speed. The first step of NGS process is to generate DNA fragments that have a size and both extremities compatible with the sequencer. The fragmentation is usually performed through either mechanical or enzymatic shearing and the quality assessed by capillary electrophoresis. Other processes such as targeted enrichment by polymerase chain reaction (PCR) are usually designed to generate molecules with a compatible size. Sequencer-specific ends are added at both extremities of every fragment by ligation of molecular adapters that are used as starting site for sequencing. These modified DNA fragments constitute a sequencing library, and usually, one library corresponds to a single sample. A molecular barcode that is made of 10–15 nucleotides is usually present in one adapter, allowing the sequencing of a mixture of libraries in a same run. The sequencing of several samples simultaneously could be then easily and safely performed, which represents a significant decrease of sequencing cost and increase of sample throughput. Despite their advanced technology, actual NGS sequencers are not sensitive enough to detect a chemical signal that would be emitted during the sequencing of a single molecule. Every molecule is amplified in close vicinity to produce a localized, uniform, and high signal intensity during sequencing. Thus, libraries are immobilized on a solid support, and clonal amplification is performed through proprietary technologies detailed hereafter. Clonally amplified and immobilized library molecules are then sequenced using sequencer-specific chemistry and strategies.

5.2.1 Illumina Sequencers

Illumina is the actual leader in the development and manufacturing of high-throughput sequencing systems. Most of public and private laboratories own one or more Illumina NGS sequencers. In 2013, Illumina sequencers represented 71 % of all installed NGS sequencers in the world. They are well known for their high-throughput sequencing data, their low error rate, and their reliability even if a lack of diversity in sequenced libraries would decrease significantly the throughput. They are actually considered as the gold standard of NGS. Illumina is an American company funded in 1998 and based in San Diego. After the successful commercialization of a bead array platform for SNP genotyping, gene expression, and protein analysis, Illumina acquired Solexa that developed the sequencing-by-synthesis technology, the technology used by all Illumina sequencers. Prepared sequencing libraries are flowed on a flow cell and are randomly immobilized through the annealing of library adapters to flow cell-coated complementary DNA fragments. Clonal amplification of each DNA molecule of the libraries is performed by bridge amplification PCR to generate isolated clusters of around one million identical single strand fragment. A sequencing primer complementary to the unbound library adapter is hybridized on almost every molecule of every cluster to start the sequencing reaction. The sequencing-by-synthesis technology uses fluorescent-labeled dNTPs that contain a terminator, which prevents the addition of several nucleotides. In every sequencing cycle, nucleotides and polymerase are flowed over the flow cell and one single dNTP is incorporated by the polymerase to each growing strand. Then, a highly sensitive camera scans the entire flow cell to detect the specific fluorescence of the dNTP added at each cluster position. The terminator is then enzymatically removed and another sequencing cycle starts. The sequence derived from every cluster that corresponds to one library molecule is then reconstituted.

The three main sequencers produced by Illumina are the HiSeqs, the MiSeq, and the NextSeq500 (Fig. 5.1) (www.illumina.com). Their price is high ranging from $750,000 for the HiSeqs to $125,000 for a MiSeq (www.allseq.com). HiSeqs are dedicated to large sequencing project such as human exome, whole genome, and transcriptome. Several HiSeq models exist. The widely used HiSeq2500 can generate up to 4 billion single reads of 125 nucleotides or paired-end reads (both extremities of library fragments sequenced) in only 5 days. It represents up to 1 terabase of sequence, enough to sequence 6 human genomes simultaneously. The HiSeq2500 can also be run in fast mode for fast turnaround sample sequencing for clinical diagnosis. It then delivers up to 1.2 billion single reads or paired-end reads of 150 nucleotides in 60 h, which represents 250–300 gigabases of sequence. Two whole human genomes can be sequenced in 60 h using this sequencer. Latest versions of HiSeq released in 2015 have an improved clustering of libraries allowing faster sequencing turnaround time and the increase of the throughput and longer reads. For example, the HiSeq4000 (2 flow cells run simultaneously) is able to generate up to 2.5 billions of up to 150 nucleotide-long reads in 3.5 days, which represents up to 750 gigabases of sequence per flow cell. The HiSeq4000 is therefore mainly dedicated to research projects, sequencing of human genomes, exomes, transcriptome, etc. To sequence human genomes with a very high throughput, two other versions of HiSeq have been released in 2014 and 2015. The HiSeq X five and the HiSeq X ten being

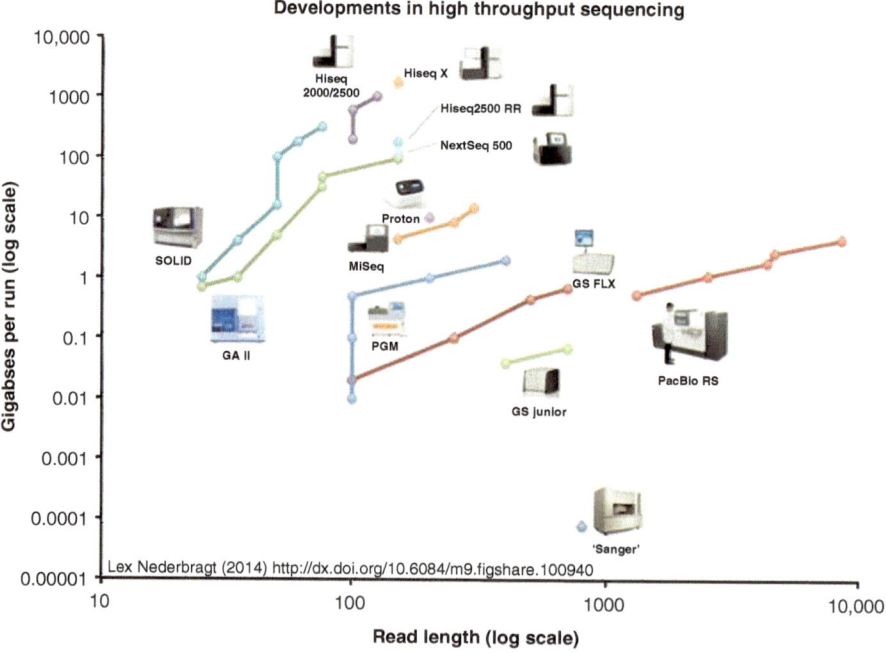

Fig. 5.1 Overview of NGS sequencers. Full run throughput in gigabases (billion bases) is plotted against single-end read length for the different sequencing platforms, both on a log scale

5 and 10 optimized and interconnected HiSeqs. The HiSeq X ten is powerful enough to sequence 18,000 human genomes in 1 year for $1,000 each, inclusive of instrument depreciation, DNA extraction, library preparation, and estimated labor for a typical high-throughput genomics laboratory. Illumina released two benchtop sequencers, the MiSeq and NextSeq500 sequencers. They are dedicated to fast sequencing and long reads with low to middle scalable throughput to match cost to sequencing data amount required. They fit perfectly the needs of the emerging sequencing-based diagnostics market. The MiSeq delivers up to 50 million single reads or paired-end reads in 55 h and with reads up to 250 nucleotides. It is mostly dedicated to targeted resequencing for clinical applications as well as for sequencing of small genomes (bacteria, yeasts) in research. The NextSeq500 delivers up to 800 million reads or paired-end reads of up to 150 nucleotides in 26 h. It is multipurpose sequencer that can sequence human exome or genome as well as small gene panels, ChIP-seq, and other mid-throughput applications.

5.2.1.1 Ion Torrent Sequencers

In 2013, Thermo Fisher Scientific bought the leader in Sanger-based sequencers Life Technologies. Life Technologies released in 2006 their first NGS sequencer, the SOLiD (Sequencing by Oligonucleotide Ligation and Detection) system and the SOLiD 5500 in 2011. Despite significant optimizations of the 5500 system, a high accuracy due to dual reading, the technology failed to move from mid high-throughput to high-throughput as Illumina successfully did. SOLiD sequencers suffered the comparison with HiSeqs because of laborious hands-on, low reliability and throughput, high cost per megabase, and lack of bioinformatics development. Life Technologies acquired then Ion Torrent Systems Inc. in 2010. Ion Torrent Systems Inc. developed an ion semiconductor sequencing technology, a method of DNA sequencing based on the detection of protons released during DNA polymerization. Development of SOLiD systems became since very limited and currently only Ion Torrent systems are sold and further developed by Thermo Fisher Scientific. Ion Torrent sequencers represented 16 % of NGS sequencers installed in the world in 2013, one fourth of Illumina sequencers. Contrary to Illumina, no fluorescence is measured during sequencing reaction but pH. First, libraries are immobilized on hydrogel beads by emulsion PCR. Briefly a single tube PCR reaction containing million of droplets each constituting a single PCR system is performed. In each droplet, one library DNA fragment and one bead are present. The library fragment hybridizes on the bead through the annealing of library adapter to complementary DNA fragments coated on. The PCR replicates more than thousand times the library molecule on the bead. Once the reaction is over, emulsion is broken and beads containing fragments are specifically recovered. This emulsion PCR-based system needs to be improved since more than one library molecule per emulsified PCR system is present in 20–30 % of droplets, leading to a loss of 20–30 % of throughput. Prepared beads are then loaded on Ion chips that are the size of a microprocessor and which contain several millions of wells; each can receive only one bead due to space limitation. This process has been recently shifted from manual to automatic with the commercialization of the Ion Chef in 2014. The ready-to-sequence chip is then loaded in an Ion Torrent sequencer, either the Ion PGM or the Ion Proton. To sequence the library molecules immobilized on beads, the sequencer flows the 4 unmodified dNTPs, dATP, dTTP, dCTP, and dGTP successively including a wash between every flow. When the flowed dNTP is complementary to the next unpaired nucleotide on the template strand, it is incorporated into the growing complementary strand by the DNA polymerase. A proton is released during this DNA polymerization, and the pH of the well in which the bead stands is modified. Each well of the chip has a corresponding ion-sensitive field-effect transistor that measures ion concentration in solution. The sequencer detects and records the pH modification every time a nucleotide is incorporated in a well. At the end of the run, the recorded signals in every well are transformed into DNA sequence corresponding to library fragments.

The two sequencers actually available, the Ion PGM and the Ion Proton, differ only by their throughput (Fig. 5.1) (www.iontorrent.com). The number of wells present in Ion chips determines the throughput of the sequencer. Three chip formats exist for Ion PGM, 314, 316, and 318 chips that can deliver up to 0.6, 3, and 5.5 million reads of maximum 400 nucleotides in 2–7 h. The Ion Proton has only one chip available, the PI chip, the PII being planned to be released in 2015. PI chip delivers up to 82 million reads of up to 200 nucleotides in 2–4 h. These throughputs are insufficient to sequence large genomes or transcriptomes, but these two benchtop sequencers were designed for the clinical diagnosis market. Their major strengths are the cost of devices ($50,000 for a PGM and $149,000 for a Proton) (www.allseq.com), the rapid sequencing that happens in less than 1 day, a scalable throughput, and low operating prices, in part because of the absence of fluorescence. The main limitations of the system are the absence of high-throughput system and the sequencing of homopolymer regions. Contrary to Illumina sequences for which only one base can be added before signal acquisition, if the same base is repeated on a template strand, then multiple nucleotides are incorporated with the Ion Torrent technology. It leads to the release of a higher rate of protons modifying proportionally the pH. A homopolymer of two consecutive identical bases has a signal twice a single nucleotide (100 % increase) which is easy to quantify, but the difference between signals corresponding to 8 and 9 identical successive nucleotides does not differ enough (theoretical increase of 12.5 %) to avoid miscalling. A lot of work is done by Ion Torrent to improve the accuracy of homopolymer sequencing, notably with the recent release of the Hi-Q chemistry.

5.2.1.2 Roche Sequencers

Roche was acquired in 2007 454 Life Sciences, a company founded by Jonathan Rothberg, the founder of Ion Torrent. The high-throughput sequencing technology developed by 454 Life Sciences is based on pyrosequencing technology and is very similar to Ion Torrent technology, but instead of pH modification, fluorescence is emitted upon nucleotide incorporation during DNA polymerization. Libraries are prepared similarly than with Ion Torrent method, and prepared beads are loaded on a Pico TiterPlate, a fiber-optic chip, one bead per well. A cocktail of enzymes, DNA polymerase, ATP sulfurylase, luciferase, and apyrase is added in every well as well as their substrates, adenosine 5' phosphosulfate (APS) and luciferin. Similarly to Ion Torrent sequencing devices, the 4 nucleotides are sequentially flowed by the sequencer into the chip, and their incorporation generates a signal recorded by the sequencer. When a nucleotide is incorporated to the growing complementary strand of a library molecule by the DNA polymerase, a pyrophosphate is released in the well. The ATP sulfurylase presents in the well converts this pyrophosphate in ATP in the presence of adenosine 5' phosphosulfate. Through the action of luciferase, luciferin is converted in oxyluciferin that generates an amount of fluorescence proportional to the amount of ATP that corresponds to the number of nucleotides incorporated. Unincorporated nucleotides as well as ATP are then degraded by the apyrase, and another nucleotide is flowed into the chip. At the end of the run, nucleotide sequence of library molecules present in every well is reconstituted. The first 454 sequencer released in 2005 was the Genome Sequencer FLX, and a newer version was released in 2008, the GS FLX + Titanium system (Fig. 5.1) (www.454. com). The last system version generates up to one million reads of up to 1000 bases in 23-h runs for a throughput of 700 megabases (www.allseq.com). This throughput is significantly lower than other sequencers on the market, but the long reads produced make this platform extremely useful for niche applications such as the assembly of *de novo* sequenced genomes. Later on a less powerful version of the Genome Sequencer FLX system, the GS Junior was released. This device can sequence up to 100,000 reads of up to 700 bases in 10 h and is mainly dedicated to researchers with modest sequencing needs. Due to a high cost per base, a high error rate in homopolymers, and low throughput compared to Illumina and Ion Torrent sequencers, Roche announced in 2013 the shutting down of their sequencing business.

5.2.1.3   The Third Generation of Sequencers

The actual second generation of sequencers suffers from bias and limitations mainly due to the requirement of amplification of library molecules before sequencing. Indeed, the signal (fluorescence, pH) detected by the sensor systems of sequencers needs to be intense to be detected. Since nucleotide incorporation does not happen correctly in all molecules of the same cluster or beads, dephasing of sequencing signal occurs along with the growing of sequenced strand and prevents the sequencing of accurate longer reads. Short reads produced by actual sequencers are not sufficient to generate long continuous assemblies of complex genomes that contain numerous repetitive sequences (transposable elements, high copy genes, centromeric/telomeric sequences, segmental duplications). The third-generation sequencers aim to be able to sequence single molecules allowing direct sequencing of nucleic acids, long reads, no bias due to amplification (GC content), and absolute quantification. Currently, only one third-generation sequencer has been released yet, the PacBio RS by Pacific Biosciences in 2010 and, its latest version, the PacBio RS II in 2013 (Fig. 5.1) (www.pacificbiosciences.com). It can generate reads of up to 15,000 bases in real time but with a reduced throughput of 50,000 reads (up to 1 gigabase sequenced) in up to 240-min run and with a much lower quality compared to second-generation sequencers. Latest version of reagents, protocol of library preparation, and system produce reads with an average length >10 kilobases (www.allseq.com). The optical system that records the sequencing signal is essentially taking a movie of fluorescent nucleotide incorporation. Briefly, single molecule is bound to a single DNA polymerase coated in a zero-mode waveguide (ZMW) on a sequencing small plastic cell called single-molecule real-time cell. ZMW is a structure that captures signal only from nucleotides that are being incorporated, while signal emitted by unincorporated is filtered out. The main applications of this system are for applications that required long reads such as de novo sequencing of small genomes. The rate of nucleotide incorporation is 2–3 bases per second, and the measure of nucleotide incorporation rate allows the determination of modification status of the template nucleotide (5-mC, 5-hmC, etc.), making this sequencer interesting for epigenetic studies. Advantages are low cost of run and single-molecule sequencing, but the main weaknesses are a high machine cost, a low throughput, and low raw accuracy of reads even if contrary to second generation of sequencers; sequencing errors are stochastic and the use of multiple reads gives high accurate consensus reads.

One of the most promising types of third-generation sequencers is based on nanopores. Several companies such as Illumina and Roche are developing or have interest in nanopore-based sequencers. Actually, the most advanced project is conducted by Oxford Nanopore Technologies, a UK-based company that has worked on nanopores for almost 20 years. In 2013, they selected genomic centers to evaluate the technology of their first nanopore-based sequencer, the MinION, which is the size of a USB key (www.nanoporetech.com). It contains biological pores through which DNA molecules pass. It is able to identify bases of DNA by measuring the changes they generate in electrical conductivity when the DNA strands flow through the pore. Sample preparation protocol includes the incorporation of a hairpin adapter that links the 2 strands of DNA molecule by one end. Both strands of a DNA molecule can be sequenced sequentially to generate a highly accurate consensus sequence. After numerous improvements of flow cells and sample preparation kits in 2014, latest released data showed that the MinION could deliver reads with a length up to 150 kilobases with an average of ~5 kilobases (Madoui et al. 2015). Some runs have produced up to 490 megabases of sequence in 48 h. The accuracy remains poor with an average identity (how closely the read matches a reference) of 75–85 % (Madoui et al. 2015). Nanopores are more than a single base in height so that the ionic signal measurements are not of individual nucleotides but of approximately 5 nucleotides at a time. Therefore, the base calling must individually recognize at least $4^5 = 1024$ possible states of ionic current for each possible 5 mer, increasing dramatically the complexity of the signal. Two other nanopore-based sequencers are currently in development by Oxford Nanopore Technologies with increase throughput, the GridION, and the PromethION which are planned to generate 1 gigabase of sequence per minute.

Several other third-generation sequencers are currently in development, notably the GnuBIO system (Bio-Rad), NabSys sequencer, GeneReader (Qiagen), etc. Some of these systems should revolutionize sequencing as NGS did and consequently genomic scientific research as well as clinical genetic testing with very fast and cheap and reliable sequencing of long DNA pieces.

5.2.2 NGS Applications

5.2.2.1 Genomics

Recent progress in technology led to substantial cost reduction and increased throughput and accuracy of DNA sequencing. A flow of genetic data has continuously grown, and scientists across many fields have used NGS for a multitude of applications (Fig. 5.2). In genomics, sequencing and resequencing of full genomes require a lot of sequencing data but few preparation steps. DNA is extracted and sheared through mechanical or enzymatic action. The library preparation consists in end repair and adapter ligation. A human genome requires at least 100 gigabases of sequences, and smaller genomes such as Escherichia coli require as little as 125 megabases that represents a tiny fraction of the NGS throughput. Sequencing a whole genome is not a standard approach even today for research or clinical applications because of its associated cost despite a huge decrease over the last 7 years. For example, tumor samples are heterogeneous, and standard genome sequencing

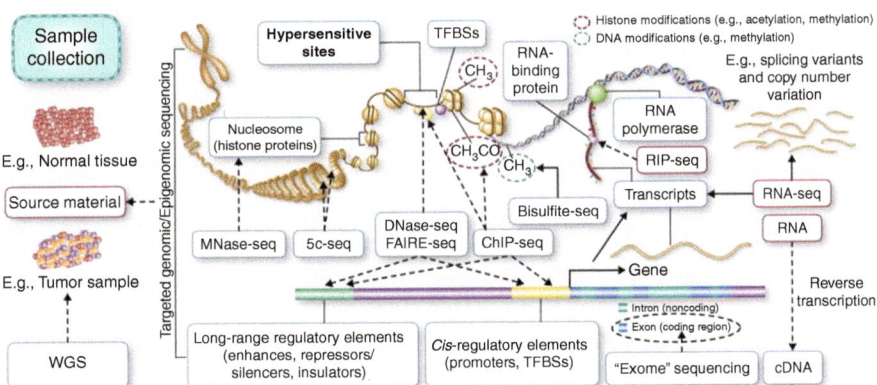

Fig. 5.2 NGS applications. WGS: whole genome sequencing; Mnase-seq: sequencing of nucleosome-associated DNA; 5c-seq (also 4C-seq, HiC-seq): chromosome conformation capture, identification of genome-wide regulatory interactions of a given locus with its unknown partners; DNAse-seq, FAIRE-seq: identification of open chromatin regions; ChIP-seq: identification of protein binding sites; Bisulfite-seq: identification of methylated regions, RIP-seq: identification of protein-RNA binding sites

used for organism genomes does not produce enough data to have a clear picture of tumor-associated molecular events. The depth of coverage which represents the number of time any targeted base is sequenced by independent sequencing reads needs to be around 100×, whereas constitutive genomes are commonly sequenced with a depth of 30×. Therefore, comprehensive sequencing of a tumor genome would cost at least 3 times more.

An alternative is the sequencing of the exome, which represents 1 % of the genome and encompasses all coding regions, or the sequencing of several genes, one gene, or a part of gene. Such targeted sequencing is achieved through the enrichment of the region of interest during library preparation before sequencing. This strategy has a reduced cost compared to the genome and allows deeper investigation of the region of interest even if the targeting strategy could be expensive depending on the method. Enrichment of targeted regions is mainly performed following two different approaches, capture and PCR amplification (Mamanova et al. 2010). The capture method is mostly used for large targets such as the exome or more than 10 genes. After library preparation, library molecules are incubated with probes designed to hybridize with targeted genomic regions. After incubation, DNA-probe complexes are recovered usually by using streptavidin-coated beads that selectively bind the biotin linked to the probes. Thus, the sequenced libraries contain only the targets. A large cumulative size of targets can be sequenced through this method, but the capture of small targets often leads to a significant portion of off-target sequencing data. Main challenges of this method are the DNA's high quality which could be challenging for some samples, long library preparation compared to other NGS applications, and specificity of the capture. Indeed, some thermodynamic constraints prevent from an efficient capture of some genomic regions (high or low GC content, repetitive regions) that lead to poor sequencing of these targets.

Isolation of regions of interest by PCR is usually the preferred method for small size cumulative target length. DNA is mixed with primers that are complimentary to regions of interest. Simultaneous amplification of all regions is performed with the multiplexing of all PCR reactions in one or more reaction tubes. Then, starting from amplified fragments, a library is prepared and sequenced. The main advantages of this technique are the ease of sample preparation and the low amount of DNA required. Furthermore, bad quality samples such as FFPE samples can be successfully processed by reducing the size of PCR products and increasing the number of primers. The main challenge of this approach is the uniformity of sequencing. Indeed, usually hundreds of PCR reactions simultaneously occur, depending on the size of the target, and since efficiency of each PCR reaction is usually nonequal, some targeted regions are poorly sequenced and some highly sequenced. This amplification heterogeneity amplifies along with the number of targets. The under- and over-sequencing has a huge impact on the final cost since the depth of sequencing wanted must be based on the poorest sequenced region. Similarly to capture method some challenging regions could neither be amplified nor sequenced. Other methods for targeted sequencing exist such as the Haloplex approach. It consists in the capture and amplification of targeted regions of DNA sheared through a constant pattern with specific cocktail of enzymes and using existing probes selected in a catalog. To help customers, exome and some predesigned gene panels have been optimized by manufacturers and can be purchased directly. Custom designs are set up through user-friendly web interface directly on manufacturer websites such as Agilent (SureSelect, Haloplex), Illumina (TruSeq, Nextera custom), and Thermo Fisher (AmpliSeq).

In addition to sequence one or more targeted genomic regions and through its quantitative properties, NGS could be used to assess copy number variants, rearranged tumoral genomes, as well as any structural and numerical chromosomal abnormalities. Data have shown that using sequencing data from exome or even from fewer targets as well as a set of control samples, a complete view of copy number variants in every targeted region for a sample can be produced (Krumm et al. 2012). Hence, NGS avoids the use of complementary experiments to get a comprehensive view of the genome studied, reducing cost and sample use. Another strategy called mate-pair sequencing allows the full study of rearrangements such as translocation using few sequencing power and therefore reduced cost (Korbel et al. 2007). It relies on the sequencing of both extremities of long DNA fragments (usually 5–15 kilobases). Through the comparison of the expected and experimentally determined distances between the two sequenced extremities, genomic structural rearrangements such as large insertion/deletions and translocations can be identified. The fragment length produced for mate-pair sequencing experiment can be experimentally tuned to change the resolution of the analysis and the final cost of the experiment.

5.2.2.2 Transcriptomics

Formerly, RNA expression was performed by quantitative PCR and then by microarray techniques. Quantitative PCR is limited since it cannot be used for whole transcriptome analysis, and microarrays suffer from reduced dynamic range. Next-generation sequencing offers rapid high-throughput gene expression profiling and any RNA type (mRNA, ncRNA, miRNa, piRNA, snRNA, etc.). Despite microarrays still being considered by many as the gold standard for genome-wide expression study, recent data have shown that NGS has a better sensitivity and has started to become the new reference tool for RNA studies since both expression quantification and sequencing can be achieved within a single experiment (Wang et al. 2009; Ledford 2008).

Depending on RNA type studied, library preparation varies. For the sequencing of mRNA transcripts, RNA should be of high quality and not fragmented. First, either mRNA is enriched using beads coated with polydT primers or a depletion of ribosomal RNA is performed. Through the use of polydT primer, only mRNAs are enriched, whereas using ribodepletion, any long RNA molecule will be sequenced, which could increase the experimental noise. PolydT-mediated enrichment is only recommended with high-quality samples since a low representation of 5' end of RNA molecule could be observed with fragmented RNA samples. RNA is then fragmented, a reverse transcription is performed to produce double-stranded cDNA fragments, and adapters are ligated at both ends. More than 100 million pairs of reads are recommended for a full human transcriptome to study expression, sequence of expressed transcripts, isoforms, as well as rearrangements (fusion, translocation). A study restricted to gene expression quantification requires as few as five million of single reads. RNA studies are usually scaled depending on the resolution needed. To sequence small RNA molecules such as miRNA, long adapters are linked directly onto the miRNA at the beginning to reach a length compatible with library preparation specifications.

The main challenge of RNA sequencing by NGS is that contrary to genomic sequencing, no standards for data control exist. Depending on sample type, the set of genes expressed varies as well as their expression. It is therefore almost impossible to control the quality of results. Synthetic RNAs could be added to the RNA sample before library preparation to evaluate biases linked to library preparation and the resolution of sequenced data. Another actual challenge of RNA sequencing is the analysis of alternative transcripts. Production of small reads by NGS sequencers complicates the characterization of all alternative transcripts even if paired-end reads have improved such analysis. Third generation of sequencers would ease the analysis of alternative transcripts through the production of long reads.

Recently, targeted RNA sequencing was developed to specifically sequence some transcripts or part of transcripts. After reverse transcription of RNA sample, a PCR is performed to enrich specifically for targeted regions. Similarly, detection of gene fusion using pre-designed mix of PCR primer can be achieved.

5.2.2.3 Other Applications

NGS has been found to be a very powerful tool to study protein-nucleic acid interactions. Chromatin immunoprecipitation followed by sequencing (ChIP-seq) is the most widely use procedure to detect the interaction between proteins and DNA (Park 2009). This technique allows researchers to identify across a whole genome binding sites of a protein of interest that can be transcription factors, DNA-binding enzymes, histones, chaperones, or nucleosomes. Chromatin-bound proteins are cross-linked and the chromatin is sheared. Chromatin fragments linked to the protein of interest are then immunoprecipitated through the use of a specific antibody. After removing nonbound chromatin, de-cross-linking step removes protein to DNA fragments that undergo library preparation and sequencing. Binding sites of the protein of interest are detected by mapping of the sequencing reads on the reference genome. Similarly, RIP-seq (RNA immunoprecipitation) is used to study RNA-protein interaction through a similar process that includes a reverse transcription to convert recovered RNA fragments in cDNA before library preparation. Compared to ChIP-chip assays (ChIP followed by microarray analysis), NGS has a better resolution, low noise, and high genomic coverage.

ChIP-seq is also used for the analysis of histone modifications that play a key role in transcriptional regulation. Active and inactive transcriptional regions of the chromatine, open and compacted chromatin states, that are regulated by specific modifications of histone (methylation, acetylation) targeted by specific antibody could be identified. To analyze transcriptional regulation, several methods exist such as DNAse-seq (Song and Crawford 2010), FAIRE-seq (Hesselberth et al. 2009), and MNase-seq (Barski et al. 2007). DNAse-seq (DNase I hypersensitive site sequencing) sequences genomic regions hypersensitive to DNAse I that are not packed, therefore implicated in transcription regulation (promoters, enhancers, cis-regulatory elements, etc.). Briefly, chromatin is digested by DNAse I that cuts DNA in non-condensed chromatin regions. Cleaved DNA fragments are purified and, after library preparation, sequenced. Mapping of sequencing reads on reference genome allows the identification of regulatory regions. An alternative to DNAse-seq is the FAIRE-seq (Formaldehyde-Assisted Isolation of Regulatory Elements). Formaldehyde is used on chromatin to link proteins to DNA. Chromatin is sheared by sonication and purified using phenol-chloroform solution. DNA that is not linked to proteins is in the aqueous phase, whereas linked DNA is in the organic phase. DNA from aqueous phase is then recovered and sequenced, thus allowing the mapping of regulatory regions across the genome. MNase-seq (micrococcal nuclease) uses the micrococcal nuclease which digests open chromatin regions to enrich for nucleosome-associated DNA (packed regions of chromatin). Sequencing of nondigested fragments reflects protection from MNase and to transcriptionally inactive genomic regions.

Another aspect of epigenetics is the study of the methylation state of DNA. Methylation occurs at CG sites through the addition of a methyl group to the cytosine by DNA methyltransferase. Methylation occurs usually in promoter regions, and the more methylated a promoter region is, the more the expression of the gene is repressed. Methylation pattern is important for embryonic development and cell differentiation. Genome-wide analysis of methylation can be achieved by bisulfite sequencing (Krueger et al. 2012) or meDIP-seq (Ruike et al. 2010), for example. Bisulfite sequencing uses the property of bisulfite to convert non-methylated cytosines into uracil while methylated cytosines are not affected. Sequencing by NGS of whole bisulfite-converted genome is challenging since the low sequence diversity complicates the mapping of reads on the reference genome since the vast majority of cytosines are sequenced as thymines after bisulfite treatment. Bisulfite is the common method to generate a clear picture of the methylome, but it is expensive, about 1.5× the cost of a genome. To lower costs, MeDIP-seq (methylated DNa immunoprecipitation) can be used as an alternative. Methylated DNA is immunoprecipitated with an antibody specific to 5'-methylcytosine. This enrichment of methylated DNA fragments does not alter genomic sequence but introduced some biases. It significantly reduces the sequencing throughput required as well as experimental cost while offering genome-wide coverage of methylation.

5.3 Challenges for the Future

Next-generation sequencing has revolutionized the field of genomics for the last 10 years. Sequencing of whole genomes or transcriptomes, large sample sets in short turnaround time, and reasonable cost have had a huge impact on scientific research and clinical genetic testing. Nevertheless, the actual second generation of sequencers suffers from limitations and biases that need to be fixed in order to get at least one gold standard technology. The huge reduction in cost has spawned an increasing demand of sequencing so that now scientist can expand sequencing targets with the ultimate goal to sequence only genomes. Targeted sequencing suffers from bias and incomplete coverage of targets as soon as a significant cumulative size of target reached a certain level. Many improvements happened with PCR-free preparation of libraries or low amount of starting material, but these types of library preparations are expensive and introduced non-PCR-based biases. The genome appears to be the next gold standard for genomics research as well as for clinical genetic testing to get a complete picture of someone's genetic background with a minimum of experimental bias. A significant step in this direction has been recently made with the \$1000 human genome cost, but another challenge has appeared: the bioinformatics capacity to treat and store such amount of sequencing data. A human genome takes roughly 1 day to be analyzed. A huge increase of genome sequencing would require a strong improvement of bioinformatics softwares to reduce calculus time and storage. It would not be surprising that costs linked to bioinformatics and storage would become similar or even higher than the cost of the sample preparation and sequencing.

The emerging third generation of sequencers shows promising early performances and gives insight to the close future of sequencing. Long reads of ten to hundreds of kilobases would help the assembly of genomes and to get a clear picture of transcriptome. Long sequencing would also improve the detection of large deletion, insertion, and chromosomal rearrangements that are of great importance for diagnostics, for example, in oncology, but still remain challenging today. Reduced error rate will also help scientific research and clinical genetic testing to avoid cross-validation and increase specificity and sensitivity of tests. Detection of variants with low frequency levels (<0.5 %) that have an interest in oncology, for example, subclonal tumoral events that could generate treatment-resistant tumor relapses, would be improved. Similarly, tracking circulating tumoral DNA would benefit patients.

References

1000 Genomes Project Consortium, Abecasis GR, Altshuler D et al (2010) A map of human genome variation from population-scale sequencing. Nature 467(7319):1061–1073. doi:10.1038/nature09534

Barski A, Cuddapah S, Cui K et al (2007) High-resolution profiling of histone methylations in the human genome. Cell 129:823–837

Bennett NC, Farah CS (2014) Next-generation sequencing in clinical oncology: next steps towards clinical validation. Cancers (Basel) 6(4):2296–2312. doi:10.3390/cancers6042296

Berkman PJ, Lai K, Lorenc MT et al (2012) Next-generation sequencing applications for wheat crop improvement. Am J Bot 99(2):365–371. doi:10.3732/ajb.1100309

Bianchi DW et al (2012) Genome-wide fetal aneuploidy detection by maternal plasma DNA sequencing. Obstet Gynecol 119(5):890–901

Bianchi DW et al (2014) DNA sequencing versus standard prenatal aneuploidy screening. N Engl J Med 370(9):799–808

Devers PL, Cronister A, Ormond KE et al (2013) Noninvasive prenatal testing/noninvasive prenatal diagnosis: the position of the National Society of Genetic Counselors. J Genet Couns 22(3):291–295. doi:10.1007/s10897-012-9564-0

Dondorp W, de Wert G, Bombard Y et al (2015) Non-invasive prenatal testing for aneuploidy and beyond: challenges of responsible innovation in prenatal screening. Summary and recommendations. Eur J Hum Genet doi:. doi:10.1038/ejhg.2015.56

Farrer RA, Kemen E, Jones JDG et al (2009) De novo assembly of the pseudomonas syringae pv. syringae B728a genome using illumina/solexa short sequence reads. FEMS Microbiol Lett 291:103–111

Hesselberth JR, Chen X, Zhang Z et al (2009) Global mapping of protein–DNA interactions in vivo by digital genomic footprinting. Nat Methods 6:283–289

http://news.thermofisher.com/press-release/life-technologies/thermo-fisher-scientific-announces-listing-ion-pgm-dx-system-us-fda-

http://pediseq.research.chop.edu/

http://www.fda.gov/NewsEvents/Newsroom/PressAnnouncements/ucm375742.htm

https://www.genome.gov/10001772

https://www.genome.gov/sequencingcosts/

International Human Genome Sequencing Consortium (2001) Initial sequencing and analysis of the human genome. Nature 409:860–921

International Human Genome Sequencing Consortium (2004) Finishing the euchromatic sequence of the human genome. Nature 431:931–945. doi:10.1038/nature03001

Korbel JO, Urban AE, Affourtit JP et al (2007) Paired-end mapping reveals extensive structural variation in the human genome. Science 318(5849):420–426

Krueger F, Kreck B, Franke A et al (2012) DNA methylome analysis using short bisulfite sequencing data. Nat Methods 9(2):145–151. doi:10.1038/nmeth.1828

Krumm N, Sudmant PH, Ko A et al (2012) Copy number variation detection and genotyping from exome sequence data. Genome Res 22:1525–1532. doi:10.1101/gr.138115.112

Lebofsky R, Decraene C, Bernard V et al (2015) Circulating tumor DNA as a non-invasive substitute to metastasis biopsy for tumor genotyping and personalized medicine in a prospective trial across all tumor types. Mol Oncol 9(4):783–790. doi:10.1016/j.molonc.2014.12.003

Ledford H (2008) The death of microarrays? Nature 455(7215):847. doi:10.1038/455847a

Lianos GD, Mangano A, Cho WC et al (2015) Circulating tumor DNA: new horizons for improving cancer treatment. Future Oncol 11(4):545–548. doi:10.2217/fon.14.250

Lo YMD, Corbetta N, Chamberlain PF et al (1997) Presence of fetal DNA in maternal plasma and serum. Lancet 350:485–487

Madoui MA, Engelen S, Cruaud C et al (2015) Genome assembly using Nanopore-guided long and error-free DNA reads. BMC Genomics 16(1):327

Mamanova L, Coffey AJ, Scott CE et al (2010) Target-enrichment strategies for next-generation sequencing. Nat Methods 7(2):111–118. doi:10.1038/nmeth.1419

Margulies M, Egholm M, Altman WE et al (2005) Genome sequencing in microfabricated high-density picolitre reactors. Nature 437:376–380

Park PJ (2009) ChIP-seq: advantages and challenges of a maturing technology. Nat Rev Genet 10(10):669–680

Rabbani B, Mahdieh N, Hosomichi K et al (2012) Next-generation sequencing: impact of exome sequencing in characterizing Mendelian disorders. J Hum Genet 57:621–632

Ruike Y, Imanaka Y, Sato F et al (2010) Genome-wide analysis of aberrant methylation in human breast cancer cells using methyl-DNA immunoprecipitation combined with high-throughput sequencing. BMC Genomics 11:137. doi:10.1186/1471-2164-11-137

Sánchez-Quinto F, Lalueza-Fox C (2015) Almost 20 years of Neanderthal palaeogenetics: adaptation, admixture, diversity, demography and extinction. Philos Trans R Soc Lond B Biol Sci 370(1660):20130374. doi:10.1098/rstb.2013.0374

Sanger F, Nicklen S, Coulson AR (1977) Proc Natl Acad Sci U S A 74(12):5463–5467

Shyr D, Liu Q (2013) Next generation sequencing in cancer research and clinical application. Biol Proced Online 15(1):4. doi:10.1186/1480-9222-15-4

Song L, Crawford GE (2010) DNase-seq: a high-resolution technique for mapping active gene regulatory elements across the genome from mammalian cells. Cold Spring Harb Protoc 2010(2):pdb.prot5384

Thomas T, Gilbert J, Meyer F (2012) Metagenomics – a guide from sampling to data analysis. Microb Inform Exp 2(1):3. doi:10.1186/2042-5783-2-3

Wang Z, Gerstein M, Snyder M (2009) RNA-Seq: a revolutionary tool for transcriptomics. Nat Rev Genet 10(1):57–63. doi:10.1038/nrg2484

Wang et al (2013) Gestational age and maternal weight effects on fetal cell-free DNA in maternal plasma. Prenatal Diagnosis 33(7):662-6

Waterston RH, Lander ES, Sulston JE (2002) On the sequencing of the human genome. Proc Natl Acad Sci U S A 99(6):3712–3716

www.454.com

www.allseq.com

www.illumina.com

www.iontorrent.com

www.nanoporetech.com/

www.pacificbiosciences.com

Chapter 6
Bioinformatics for Precision Medicine in Oncology

Nicolas Servant and Philippe Hupé

6.1 Data Integration Challenges and Solutions

This section is based on the open access article written by Servant et al. (2014).

6.1.1 Framework for Precision Medicine in Oncology

Precision medicine requires a strong interdisciplinary collaboration between several stakeholders covering a large continuum of expertise ranging from medical, clinical, biological, translational, technical, and biotechnological know-hows. Figure 6.1 illustrates the different practitioners involved in the complex process, describes the data workflow starting from and coming back to the patient in order to tailor the therapy, and shows the informatics and bioinformatics infrastructure supporting the workflow. To build the therapeutic decision, the most exhaustive data ranging from clinical to biological, environmental, and family information (e.g., description of the tumor histology, list of previous treatments, family history, etc.) needs to be collected along a complex healthcare pathway. As the disease evolves, new experiments such as high-throughput screens (e.g., with microarray or NGS technologies) or biomarkers detection by immunohistochemistry (IHC) have to be performed to

N. Servant (✉)
Bioinformatics Platform, Institut Curie, Paris, France

Unité INSERM/Institut Curie U900, Paris, France
e-mail: nicolas.servant@curie.fr

P. Hupé, PhD
Bioinformatics Platform, Institut Curie, Paris, France
e-mail: philippe.hupe@curie.fr

© Springer International Publishing Switzerland 2015
C. Le Tourneau, M. Kamal (eds.), *Pan-cancer Integrative Molecular Portrait Towards a New Paradigm in Precision Medicine*,
DOI 10.1007/978-3-319-22189-2_6

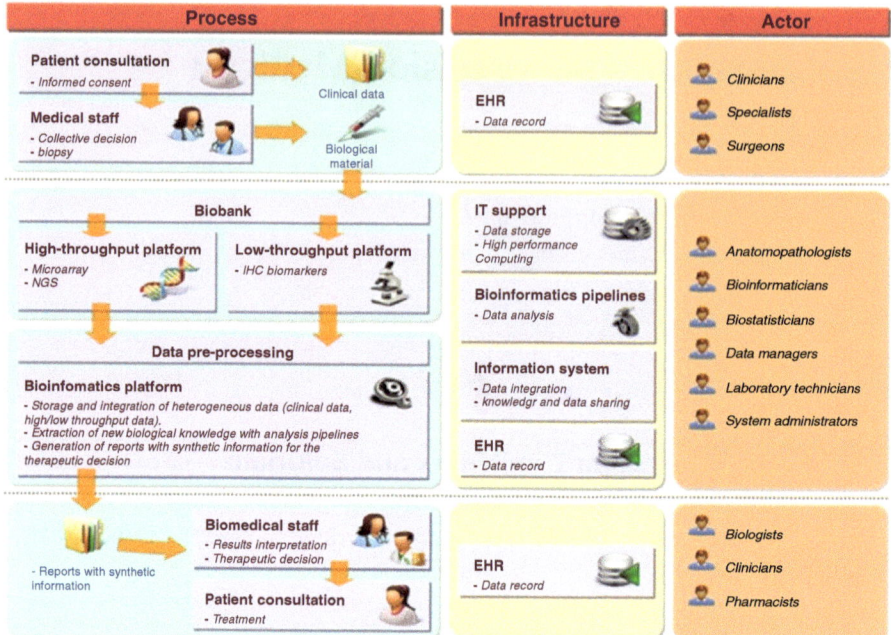

Fig. 6.1 Framework for PM in oncology. The *left part* describes the workflow and processes required for the decision-making from patient consultation to the therapeutic decision. The *middle part* focuses on the informatics and bioinformatics architecture required to support the different steps of the workflow. The *right part* indicates the different experts involved in each process

measure relevant biological information required to choose the best therapy. During the process, physicians (including different specialists such as surgeons, pathologists, radiation and medical oncologists, etc.), biologists, pharmacists, bioinformaticians, computational biologists, biostatisticians, informaticians, biobank managers, biotechnological platform managers, clinical research associates, and the technical staff will offer their expertise for the benefit of the patient. Different actors and cultures and a variety of miscellaneous constraints, including meeting the deadlines for results delivery, render the application of PM in daily clinical practice extremely challenging. Organizational aspects are therefore essential for the success of PM (Veltman et al. 2013). Downing et al. (2009) mentioned the importance of electronic health record (EHR) and clinical decision support (CDS) for care delivery due to the acceleration of knowledge discovery and its impact on the increasing number of possible clinical decisions. Development in CDS is required to handle the large heterogeneity of data and their complexity. The authors also pinpoint the fact that PM strongly depends on our ability to collect, disseminate, and process complex information. Indeed, every stakeholder produces information during the healthcare pathway at different time points and in different places. The overall information needs to be gathered, integrated, and summarized in a digest report to facilitate the therapeutic decision-making.

6.1.2 Need for Bioinformatics Solutions to Support Precision Medicine

The availability of high-throughput technologies dedicated to clinical applications makes it very attractive for cancer centers to use these new tools on a daily basis. However, establishing such a clinical facility is not a trivial task due to the afore-mentioned complexity of PM framework along with the overwhelming amount of data. Indeed, the field of oncology has entered the so-called big data era as the particle physics did several years ago. From the big data 4 V's perspective, data integration issue (i.e., merging heterogeneous data in a seamless information system) in oncology can be formulated as follows: a large *volume* of patients' data is disseminated across a large *variety* of databases which increase in size at a huge *velocity*. In order to extract most of the hidden *value* from these data, we must face challenges at (1) the technical level to develop a powerful computational architecture (software/hardware); (2) the organizational and management levels to define the procedures to collect data with highest confidence, quality, and traceability; and (3) the scientific level to create sophisticated mathematical models to predict the evolution of the disease and risks to the patient. Obviously, an efficient informatics and bioinformatics architecture is definitely needed to support PM in order to record, manage, and analyze all the information collected. The architecture must also permit the query and the easy retrieval of any data that might be useful for therapeutic decision in real time, thus allowing clinicians to propose the tailored therapy to the patient in the shortest delay. Therefore, bioinformatics is among the most important bottlenecks toward the routine application of PM, and several challenges need to be faced to make it a reality (Fernald et al. 2011). First, the development of a seamless information system allowing data integration, data traceability, and knowledge sharing across the different stakeholders is mandatory. Second, bioinformatics pipelines need to be developed in order to provide relevant biological information from the high-throughput molecular profiles of the patient. Third, the architecture must warrant the reproducibility of the results.

If many recent publications point out the key role of the bioinformatics for PM today (Simon and Roychowdhury 2013), clinical trials usually do not detail the complete bioinformatics environment used in practice to assess the quality and the traceability of the generated data. Different software platforms such as tranSMART (Athey et al. 2013), G-DOC (Madhavan et al. 2011) or the cBioPortal for Cancer Genomics (Cerami et al. 2012) have been recently developed to promote the data sharing and analysis of genomics data in translational research. Canuel et al. (2014) reviewed the different solutions available and compared their functionalities. One of the most interesting features of these platforms relies on their analytical functionalities. They provide ready-to-use tools through user-friendly interface offering interesting functionalities for data queries and user analysis. However, these different solutions do not address essential aspects which are offered by our system: first, often they handle a specific type of data; second, they do not cover management and traceability of the data in real time as long as they are generated by the different stakeholders; and third, they do not provide clinicians with a meaningful digest of the analyses, which they need to take clinical decisions.

6.1.3 Seamless Information System

Precision medicine relies on a tight connection between many different stakeholders. As the choice of the therapy is based on a combination of different information levels including clinical data, high-throughput profiles (somatic mutations and DNA copy number alterations), and IHC data, all this information related to a given patient needs to be gathered in a seamless information system. Data integration is definitely required, and bioinformatics plays a central role in setting up this infrastructure. The information system must ensure data sharing, cross software interoperability, automatic data extraction, and secure data transfer. In the context of the SHIVA clinical trial, high-throughput and IHC data are sent by the different biotechnological platforms to the bioinformatics platform using standardized procedures for transfer and synchronization. Data are then integrated into the information system within ad hoc repositories and databases. Metadata describing the data are stored in the core database such as the patient identifier, the type of data (e.g., mutation screening, clinical data, DNA copy number profile), and the technology used (e.g., Affymetrix microarray, Ion Torrent™ PGM sequencing). Each type of data is then processed by dedicated bioinformatics pipelines in order to extract the relevant biological information such as the list of mutations and the list of amplifications/deletions. Therefore, the core database of the system acts as a hub allowing referencing all data through the use of web services. It knows exhaustively which data is available for a given patient and where the raw and processed data are physically stored. It thus offers the possibility for clinicians to make queries through a web application and to extract the list of available information for a given patient. In addition, the system is also used to manage and perform automatic integrative analysis required for the therapeutic decision.

6.2 High-Throughput Data Analyses and Reporting

The DNA copy number analysis is now well defined, following standard analysis workflow. Many other books or papers already present in details this application. For this reason, the current section is mainly dedicated to NGS data analysis.

6.2.1 DNA Copy Number Analysis

The use of DNA copy number microarray allows both the detection of DNA copy number alterations and the loss of heterozygosity events. As an example, we will illustrate the analysis of Affymetrix microarray data.

Raw data are usually normalized with the Affymetrix Power Tools software package (http://www.affymetrix.com) in order to remove systematic and technological bias. Then, the log R ratio is segmented in order to detect breakpoints and assign copy number status (Rigaill 2010; Hupé et al. 2004). A similar process is applied on the allele difference profile as performed by the GAP software (Popova et al. 2009). Both profiles (DNA copy number and LOH) allow the estimation of absolute copy number for each probe taking into account the sample cellularity and tumor ploidy.

Each gene status (normal, gained, amplified, lost, deleted, loss of heterozygosity) can then be assessed. Copy number alterations are defined as follows: deletion=0 copy; loss=1 copy; normal=2 copies; gain=3, 4, or 5 copies; and amplification ≥6 copies for diploid tumor and deletion=0 copy; loss=1 or 2 copies; normal=3 or 4 copies; gain=5 or 6 copies; and amplification ≥7 copies for tetraploid tumors.

Additional steps in the analysis can be performed to distinguish between large-scale events such as chromosome arm gain and focal events targeting single onco-gene or tumor-suppressor gene. Focal gains and amplifications are defined as genomic alterations with a size less than 10 Mb and a copy number greater than the surrounding regions. In order to check whether a focal gain or an amplification of a size between 1 and 10 Mb induces a protein overexpression, a validation using IHC can be applied for clinical decision.

6.2.2 Analysis of High-Throughput Sequencing and Clinical Applications

6.2.2.1 General Principles of High-Throughput Sequencing Analysis

The next-generation sequencing (NGS) technologies have emerged around 2008 and have exploded a few years later. First used in research projects, they rapidly pave the way to new clinical applications. Today, the NGS technologies have almost no limitation in terms of biological applications and continue to evolve very rapidly. NGS offers the possibility to sequence a full human genome in less than two weeks for a few thousand dollars where 2.7 billions dollars and more than 10 years were required by the Human Genome Project to deliver the first human genome draft in 2001. In early 2004, the second generation of sequencers provided an increase of the throughput capacity with a lower cost and is today widely used both in research and clinical screenings. NGS technologies are a very competitive field and third (single molecule) and fourth generations (nanopore technologies) of sequencers are already available or under development.

The biological applications of NGS can be broadly classified in three main classes according to their biological context: the DNA world, the RNA world, and the epigenetic world, each of them being subdivided in several sequencing techniques and methodological workflows. If the use of RNA sequencing starts to emerge as a diagnosis tool, the DNA sequencing remains the main application for clinics. In addition to whole-genome sequencing, target-enrichment methods have been developed to selectively capture genomic regions of interest from a DNA sample prior to sequencing. The exome sequencing consists of selecting only the subset of DNA coding regions before sequencing. Other targeted strategies can be defined at the gene or amplicon levels, making these applications cost-effective for a large number of samples.

The analysis of these data has been an important bioinformatics challenge of the recent years. The main difficulty in comparison with the microarray analyses comes from the size of the data to manipulate. Thus, if microarray analysis can be performed today on a single laptop, analyzing a large NGS dataset requires a dedicated computational infrastructure as well as strong computational skills. Once the targeted DNA region is sequenced, the first steps of the analysis are usually common to many different types of sequencing applications (quality control, cleaning, reads alignment). Then, the secondary analysis aims at answering a dedicated biological question. In oncology, this question is usually to detect with high sensibility and specificity somatic mutations. But other questions such as detection of copy number variants or large rearrangements can also be addressed using NGS techniques. In the following part, we will describe in details each step of the analysis, from the raw reads to the list of filtered variants used by the clinicians for therapeutical decision.

6.2.2.2   Definition and Key Concepts

Before presenting the different steps of a sequencing analysis project, key notions and vocabulary common to all applications have to be defined. The reads refer to the sequences called and delivered by the sequencing machine. These reads are associated with quality values describing the probability of a given call to be a sequencing error (see Sect. 6.2.2.3 for details). The first question which usually comes when a project is designed is about the number of reads required to answer the biological question. Whereas the recent technologies are able to produce billion of reads per flow cell, most of the applications only require a few dozen (or hundred) millions of reads per sample, thus allowing the multiplexing of several samples using different barcodes. The number of reads required per sample depends on the sequencing depth, which is the average number of reads spanning one nucleotide. For instance, the current sequencing depth advised to detect with a good accuracy a germline variant is around 30X. It means that a homozygous variant should be supported in average by 30 reads (15 for each allele in the case of a heterozygous variant). In the case of somatic mutations and cancer samples, the higher will be the sequencing depth, and the lower will be the detection threshold at which a variant may be called. For instance, with a sequencing depth of 100X, a variant with a frequency of 10 % will be supported by only ten reads. Note that it is important to differentiate the sequencing depth from the coverage. The latter represents the fraction of the genome which is supported by at least one read (Fig. 6.2).

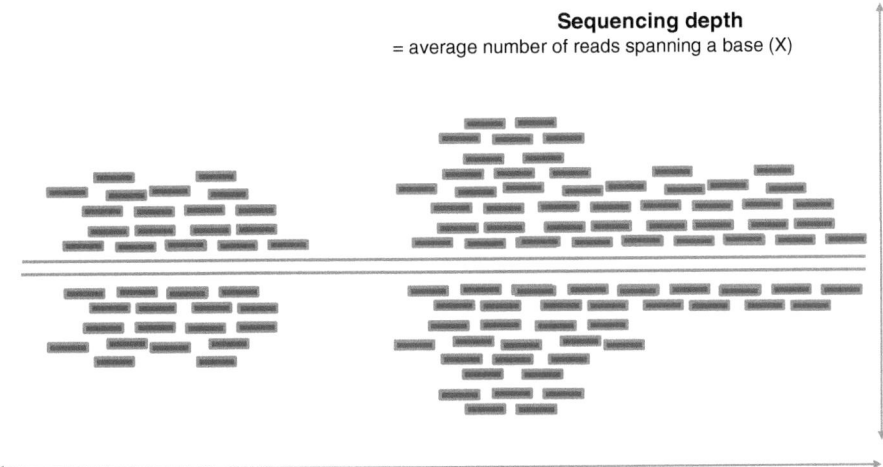

Fig. 6.2 Sequencing depth *versus* coverage. The sequencing depth is defined as the mean number of reads covering one base, whereas the coverage represents the fraction of the genome which is read at least once

6.2.2.3   Quality Control of Sequencing Reads

Any high-throughput technology, even if well standardized, suffers from experimental bias. Adequate experimental designs and good laboratory practice are thus mandatory to limit the variation among samples. This point is even more true in clinical practice where the reliability of high-throughput screening is expected to be higher. Therefore, a quality control procedure needs to be defined.

The *FASTQ* format is a standard text-based format for storing both the nucleotide sequence and its corresponding quality scores. Both the nucleotide and the quality score at each position are encoded as ASCII character. The quality values are encoded as Phred scores Q and are logarithmically related to the base-calling error probabilities P (1):

$$Q = -10 \log 10 P\left(1\right)$$

For instance, a Phred quality score of 20 (Q20) assigned to a base means that the probability of an incorrect base call is 1–100 times (Table 6.1). It means that the base call accuracy is 99 % and that every 100 bp, a sequencing read will likely contain an error.

Table 6.1 Phred quality value

Phred quality score	Error probability	Base accuracy (%)
10	1 in 10	90
20	1 in 100	99
30	1 in 1000	99.9
40	1 in 10,000	99.99

The sequencing quality values are encoded as Phred scores and are logarithmically related to the base-calling error probabilities. A minimum quality score of 20 is usually used to select high confidence data.

Starting from the raw reads from the sequencers, several quality controls can be applied:

1. *Sequence quality.* One standard way of representing the reads quality is to display the range of quality values across all bases at each position in the FASTQ file. The first nucleotides of the reads usually have a very good quality which tends to decrease with the size of the sequence. A good sequencing run is expected to have quality scores all above 20 (or even 30). If the quality drops below this level after a certain point along the read, it might be useful to trim all reads to be shorter than that length. Another way of representing sequences quality is to look at the average quality scores per sequence. Reads with low average quality should be discarded from the dataset.

2. *Sequence content.* In practice, good sequencing runs should have no variation among base calls or GC content along the length of the reads. The base content, however, can be different from an organism to another or from an application to another. Note that an erratic behavior on the first three bases can be observed with Illumina sequencing. This is usually a random primer effect which is in practice not completely random. If the sequencer is not able to provide a base call with sufficient confidence at a given position, it will return an *N* base. An unexpected number of *N* calls at each position (higher than a few percent) can reveal a base call issue during the sequencing.

3. *Sequence length distribution.* For most sequencing technology (e.g., Illumina), the sequence length is expected to be uniform, but others can produce reads of different lengths (e.g., Life Technologies Ion Torrent). It can thus be useful to compare the relative proportion of reads with a given size and to correlate this information with the fragment size and protocol used for the library preparation.

4. *Duplicate sequences.* A good sequencing library is expected to present a large diversity of DNA fragments, corresponding to a low level of duplication. A high level of duplication is likely to indicate a sequencing bias due to PCR over amplification. Duplicates are defined as reads (or pair of reads) with exactly the same sequence, aligned at exactly the same position on the genome.

5. *Contamination and overrepresented sequences.* As for the duplication level, no overrepresented sequence is expected to be found in a good sequencing library. Note that this observation mainly depends on the application. Overrepresented sequences are more likely to be observed in targeted sequencing where, by

construction, the diversity of the library is less important. RNA sequencing can also provide overrepresented sequence according to the expression level and the size of the genes. The overrepresented sequences can also be associated with the adapter sequences used during the library preparation. Contamination can also be assessed by aligning a fraction of reads on known bacterial genomes.

Many different bioinformatics solutions have been developed for NGS quality controls. Among them, the FastQC software developed at the Babraham Institute is largely used by the community (http://www.bioinformatics.babraham.ac.uk/projects/fastqc/). All the quality controls discussed before are provided are illustrated on (Fig. 6.3).

6.2.2.4   Reads Alignment on a Reference Genome

The reads alignment (also called reads mapping) is the process of figuring out where in the genome a sequence is from. The reads alignment differs from the reads de novo assembly in the way that it is based on a known reference genome. De novo assembly strategies are usually used to reconstruct DNA contigs or RNA transcripts without reference genome. Note that some strategies have been developed using

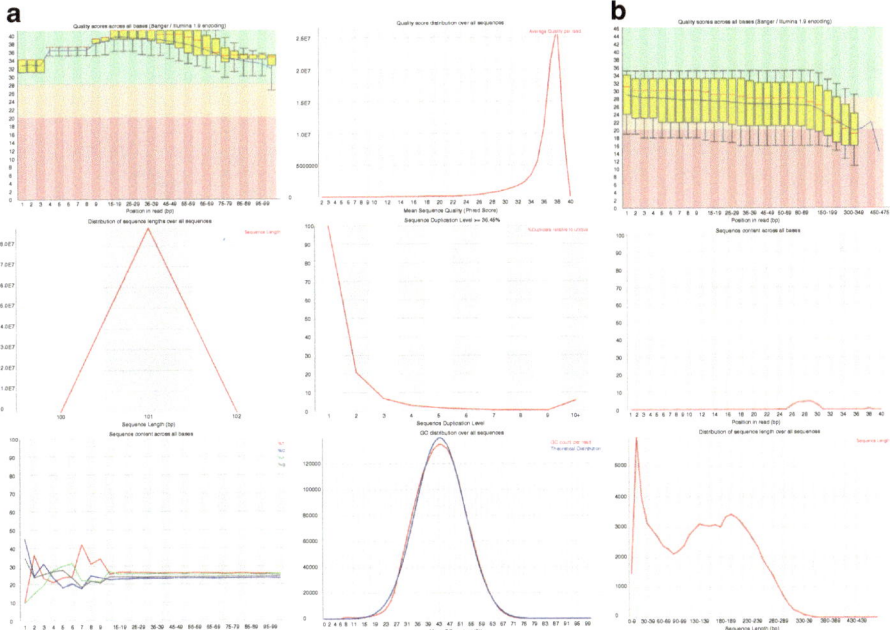

Fig. 6.3 Quality control of raw sequencing reads. (**a**) Outputs from the FastQC software showing, from top left to bottom right; quality value distribution per position; distribution of mean quality values per reads; reads length; duplicates level; base composition; GC content. (**b**) Examples of bad-quality profiles from top to bottom; low-quality values per base; fraction of N bases; reads length distribution with very small sequences

both reads mapping and reads assembly to reconstruct highly rearranged tumor genomes. In terms of complexity and time requirements, de novo assemblies are orders of magnitude slower and more memory intensive than reads alignment (Fig. 6.4).

Reads alignment can be seen as an (in)exact matching problem, i.e., given a long text and a much smaller pattern, the goal is to find the location in the text where the pattern occurs (allowing a predetermined number of misalignment).

Two main challenges have to be faced up. The first one is practical: if the reference genome is very large (3.10^9 nucleotides for the human genome) and if we have hundred of millions of reads, how quickly and efficiently is aligning these reads on the genome? The second is methodologic: sequencing errors or polymorphisms as well as reads coming from repetitive elements make the problem much more difficult in practice. In some cases, detecting the unique position on the genome where the read belongs to is impossible. If so, the program should choose to report multiple possible locations or to select one location randomly.

Understanding in details the algorithm of an alignment software is usually not necessary to use it in practice. In the following section, we will focus on the practical matters and the rationales of reads alignment.

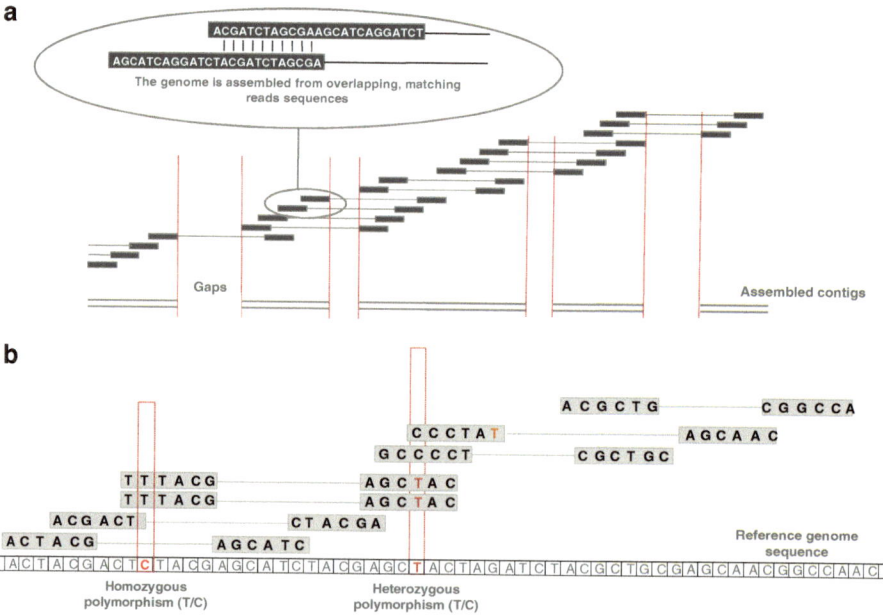

Fig. 6.4 Difference between genome assembly and reads alignment. (**a**) Reads are aligned and merged together in order to reconstruct the original sequence, usually represented as contigs. (**b**) Reads alignment on a reference genome. Misalignments can either represent a true variant information or a sequencing error

Compression and Indexes

The first step of the reads alignment is the choice of the reference genome to work with. The reference genome has to be indexed before running the alignment. Like the index of a book, the index of the reference genome allows the program to rapidly find shorter sequences embedded within it. Several strategies have been proposed to build indexes based on a data structure allowing an efficient memory storage and a rapid course of the data. The Burrows-Wheeler transform (BWT) is a compression process that reorders the genome in a way that exact repeated sequences are collapsed together in the data structure (Fig. 6.5). It is reversible, so that the original sequence can easily be reconstructed from the transform. The transformation was originally discovered by David Wheeler in 1983 and was published by Michael Burrows and David Wheeler in 1994. This method is used by popular reads alignment software, such as Bowtie (Langmead et al. 2009), Bowtie2 (Langmead and Salzberg 2012), GEM (Marco-Sola et al. 2012), and BWA (Li et al. 2009). These softwares are fast allowing the alignment of 100 millions reads in a few hours, requiring a few gigabytes of memory. The main limitation of this approach is the number of mismatches or gaps allowed in the read. However, as sequencing becomes increasingly accurate, this limitation is likely to become less important for species with relatively low polymorphism rates.

Searching

Without considering the sequencing errors, the existing polymorphisms between the reference genome and the real sequence usually require more flexible strategies allowing mismatches and gaps. In the context of oncology and DNA sequencing, allowing gaps is mandatory to detect variants and insertion/deletion events. BWT is extremely fast for finding exact alignments, whereas dynamic programming is flexible and allows gaps detection. In this way, an alignment is usually characterized by a score that reflects the global match, mismatch, and gap rates. The higher is the score, the better is the alignment. The scoring system can also used the raw Phred quality of each nucleotide. It is thus more likely to observe a true mismatch at a low Phred quality position (Fig. 6.6). Changing the scoring system of the software will change the number and quality of reads that map to the reference and the time it takes to complete the alignment. It is also important to notice that many alignment softwares are based on heuristics. This means that the reported alignment is not guaranteed to be the best one. The alignment accuracy can usually be defined but at a cost of intensive computing time.

Since sequencing technologies are now able to generate longer reads, recent alignment softwares now propose both local and global alignment strategies. Global alignment is appropriate for sequences that are expected to share similarity over their whole length, meaning that the entire read must be aligned on the reference genome, whereas local alignment is appropriate when the sequences may show isolated regions of similarity, meaning that only a subpart of the read can be aligned on

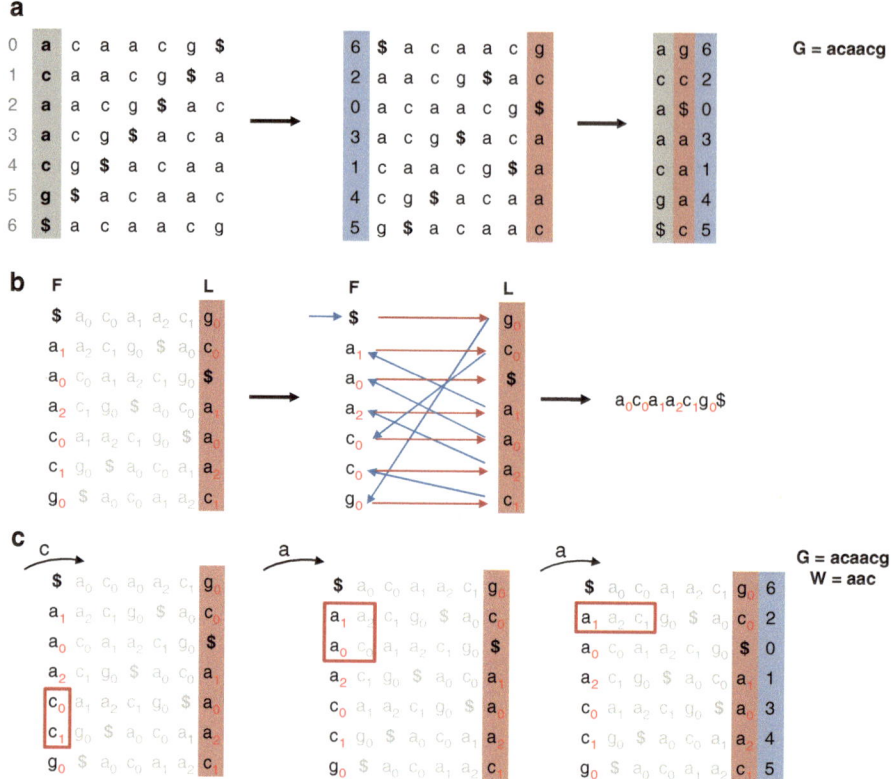

Fig. 6.5 Burrows-Wheeler transform and exact mapping. (**a**). Burrows-Wheeler transform (BWT). The BWT transformation can be achieved in three steps. First, we apply a rotation on the string G by repeatedly taking a character from one end and sticking it on the other. The rows are then sorted by alphabetical order. The final column represents the BWT transformation. (**b**) LF mapping. The BWT is reversible through LF mapping which is based on the property that the ith occurrence of a character c in the last column has the same rank as the ith occurrence of c in the first column. (**c**) Exact matching. The BWT can be used as an efficient index of G (FM-index). The matching starts by finding the rows beginning with the shortest proper suffix of W. Then, because only the F, L, and rank columns are stored in the index, the LF mapping strategy is used to extend the suffix until exact matching

the reference. The unmapped part is usually returned as soft-clipped sequence occurring at one or both ends of the read (Fig. 6.7).

Reporting

Understanding how alignment positions are reported by the software is extremely important for downstream analyses. Depending of the genome complexity and size, a large majority of reads is expected to be uniquely aligned on the reference

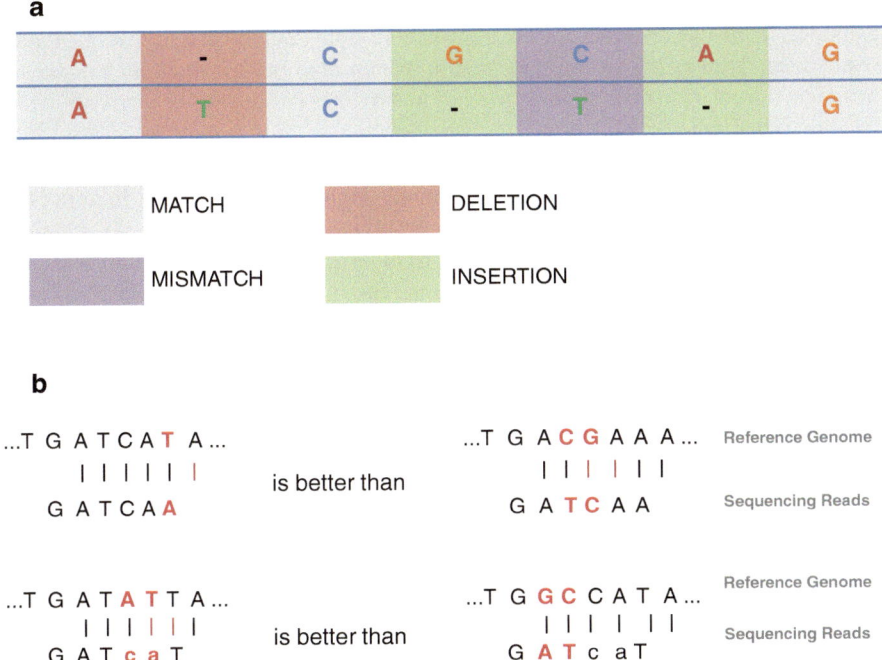

Fig. 6.6 Rationale of reads alignment. (**a**) Definition of match, mismatch, insertion, and deletion. (**b**) The goal of reads alignment is to find the best reads position in a reference sequence. In this way, allowing one mismatch is better than allowing two mismatches. In addition, reads mapper is usually able to use base quality values. Therefore, allowing two mismatches on low quality bases (lower case) is better than mismatches on high confidence bases

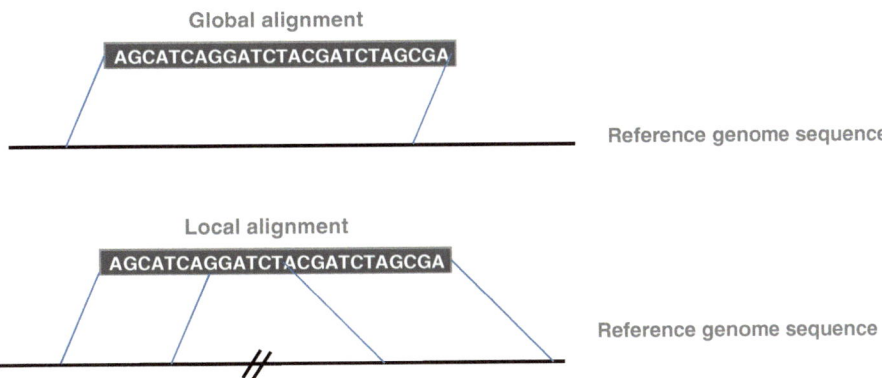

Fig. 6.7 Global *versus* local mapping strategy. Global (or end-to-end) strategy will align the entire read sequence on the reference genome. Local alignments find the best alignments of sequence segments, which can be separated and in any order

genome. Keeping only those unique reads ensures a high-quality alignment but excludes from the analysis all the repeated regions. According to the biological context, reads aligning to multiple positions can also be informative. This is, for instance, the case of reads spanning genes and their pseudogenes or reads aligned to intronic repetitive sequences.

Paired-end sequencing comes with a prior expectation about the relative orientation of the mates and the distance separating them on the original DNA fragment. In most of the case, both mates are first independently aligned on the reference genome. An additional step is thus required to pair both alignments trying to promote concordant reads pairs. A concordant read pair is defined by an expected distance between the two mates and a concordant mate orientation. Some aligner such as BWA should be able to promote a suboptimal position if its mate is hanging around. This is useful to anchor reads in repeats.

Once the alignment is performed, the mapping quality score (*MAQ*) of a given read quantifies the probability that its position on the genome is correct. The mapping quality is encoded in the Phred scale (see 1.) where *P* is the probability that the alignment is not correct.

The probability is calculated as:

$$P = 10^{(-MAQ/10)}$$

Where *MAQ* is the mapping quality. For example, a mapping quality of 40 = 10 to the power of −4, meaning that there is a 0.01 % chance that the read was aligned incorrectly.

The mapping quality is therefore associated with several alignment factors.

- *The base quality of the read.* If the base quality of the read is low, it means that the observed sequence might be wrong and thus that its alignment is wrong.
- *The complexity of the reference genome.* The mappability refers to the complexity of the genome. Repeated regions are more difficult to map, and reads falling in these regions usually get low mapping quality. In this context, the *MAQ* will reflect the fact that the reads are not uniquely aligned and that their real origin cannot be determined.
- *The paired-end information.* In case of paired-end sequencing data, concordant pairs are more likely to be well aligned.

The higher is the mapping quality, the better is the alignment. A read aligned with a good mapping quality usually means that the read sequence was good was aligned with few mismatches in a high mappability region.

The *MAQ* value can be used as a quality control of the alignment results. The proportion of reads aligned with an *MAQ* higher than 20 is usually used for downstream analyses.

Alignment Quality

Simple descriptive statistics are advised after the reads alignment. The proportion of aligned reads, the sequencing depth, and the coverage are important factors of the alignment quality (Fig. 6.8). In the case of paired-end data, the number of

Fig. 6.8 Alignment reporting of an exome sequencing. Reads coverage for one hundred exomes at different sequencing depth. In the context of exome sequencing, one can expect to have more than 80 % of the targets covered at 20× and more

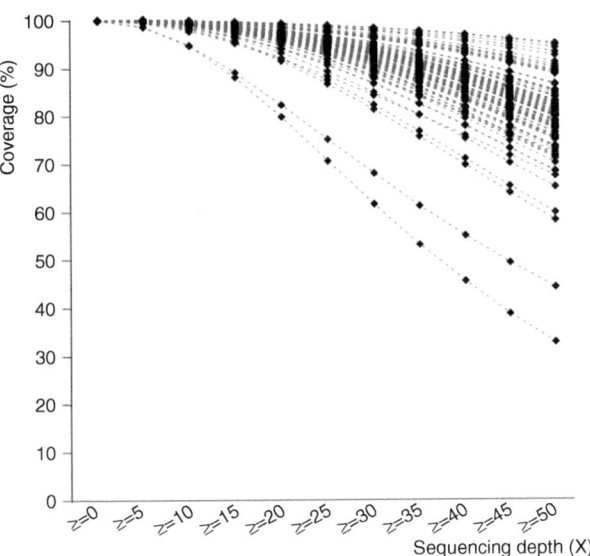

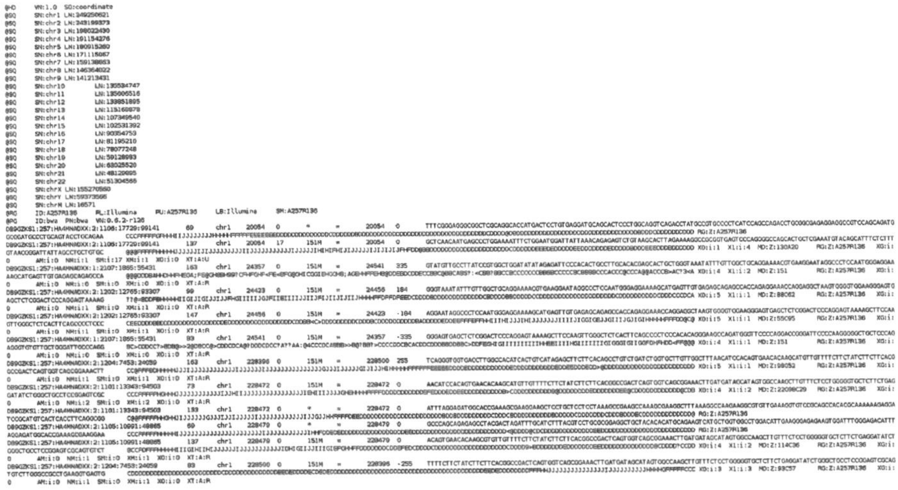

Fig. 6.9 SAM format. Example of SAM format. After the header, each row represents one read, described by its name, flag, alignment position, CIGAR, sequence, and qualities

concordant and discordant pairs is also a good indicator of the alignment quality. Apart from a specific biological context, the proportion of discordant reads pairs is expected to be low. A high number of discordant pairs should mean that the mapping was not correctly performed. Sequencing depth of sexual chromosomes can be used to validate the sex of the patients. In the case of paired samples, i.e., normal and tumor samples, it is also strongly recommended to focus on some known human SNPs and to validate the presence/absence of these SNPs in both normal and tumor samples.

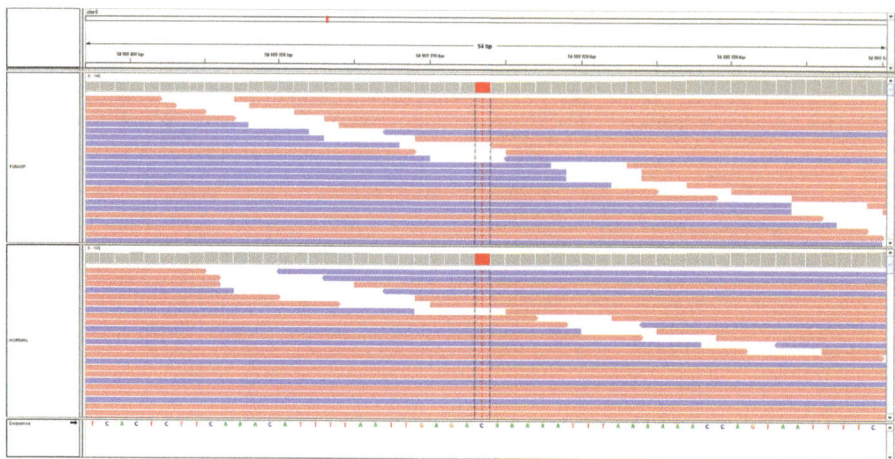

Fig. 6.10 Visualization of aligned data using the IGV software. Forward and reverse reads are, respectively, represented in *red and blue*. A homozygous variant is represented in red where a T is observed in the samples and a C is expected according to the reference genome

Alignment Format

Alignment softwares usually work with *FASTQ* files as input and deliver a *SAM* (Sequence Alignment/Map format) file as output (Li et al. 2009). The *SAM* format is now a standard to store aligned data (Fig. 6.9). The *BAM* format is the compressed binary form of the *SAM* format and is commonly used because less disk-space consuming. Each line represents a read alignment with 11 mandatory fields such as the read name, mapping position, *MAQ*, *CIGAR*, sequence, and quality sequence. The CIGAR string describes how the read is aligned. For instance, the string "35MI2M13" means that the read was aligned with 35 matches or mismatches (M), followed by an insertion (I) of 2 nucleotides and 13 matches or mismatches (M). Note that matches and mismatches are encoded with the same character M. The CIGAR string can therefore be interpreted and used by visualization software such as the IGV software (Fig. 6.10).

A flag is also added for each alignment. This flag can be used to quickly filter out the alignments with the SAMtools suite. For instance, all unmapped reads will have a flag equal to four, reads aligned on reverse strand will have a flag equal to 16, etc. Additional tags, such as the number of mismatch (@NM), the read group (@RG), the mapping quality of the mate (@MQ), etc., are also reported but can differ from an alignment software to another. Finally, note that the BAM format without alignment position data is also increasingly used as a space-saving alternative to FASTQ files for containing the short raw read data.

Post-processing

Most of the NGS analysis softwares now work with SAM/BAM files as input. Processing these files can be easily achieved using dedicated programs such as SAMtools and *Picard tools* (http://broadinstitute.github.io/picard/). SAMtools is a

Table 6.2 Reads filtering
and SAM flag

Flag	Description
4	Read is not aligned
12	Both paired-end reads are not aligned
16	Read is aligned on reverse strand
1	Read is paired
2	Read aligned in proper pair

Example of SAM flag from https://broadinstitute.
github.io/picard/explain-flags.html. Reads can be filtered using the *SAMtools* software and the -f/-F options.

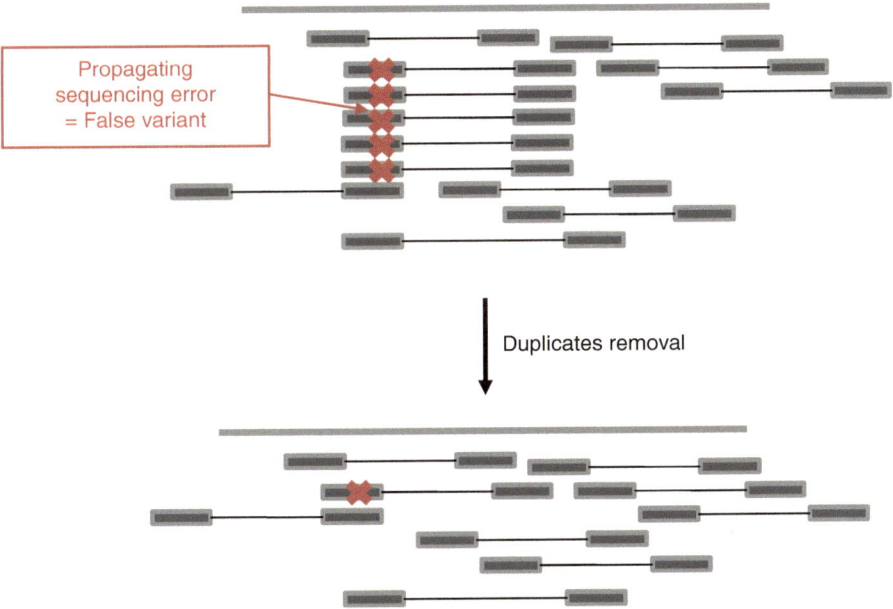

Fig. 6.11 Duplicates and PCR artifacts. Duplicates are usually artifacts due to the PCR cycles
during library preparation. Keeping duplicates for downstream analysis might lead to sequencing
error propagation and false-positive variants

popular suite of commands which allows efficiently viewing, sorting, merging, or
indexing a SAM/BAM file (Li et al. 2009). Using the flag or the MAQ described
below, SAMtools allows to filter out or to keep the alignments with the speci-
fied flag/MAQ (see Table 6.2 for examples, http://broadinstitute.github.io/picard/
explain-flags.html).

The *Picard tools* are also commonly used to process the SAM/BAM files. One of
its most powerful applications is to detect and mark/remove the duplicated reads.
Duplicates are usually defined as reads with the same start position and the same
CIGAR string. In other words, they correspond to the exact same DNA fragment. If
a few percentages of duplicates can be "biologically" expected according to the
sequencing application, most of them are usually artifacts due to the PCR cycles
during the library preparation (Fig. 6.11). For full-genome sequencing, it is therefore advice to remove the duplicates before downstream analyses. Of note, for target

sequencing, removing or not the duplicates depends of the size of the target and of the library preparation used. The smaller the targeted region, the higher the duplicates' level should be.

The quality control and the reads alignment are common steps of any bioinformatics analysis of NGS data with, of course, specificity about the reference, the parameters, or the strategy to use. On the contrary, the secondary analysis will be completely different according to the biological context and sequencing application.

6.2.2.5 Detection of Genomic Variants

Different Classes of Variants

In oncology, the detection of deleterious mutations is a recurrent question which offers a lot of different applications from the fundamental research to the choice of a treatment. A genomic variant can be classified as a single-nucleotide variant (SNV), an insertion/deletion (indel), or a structural variant.

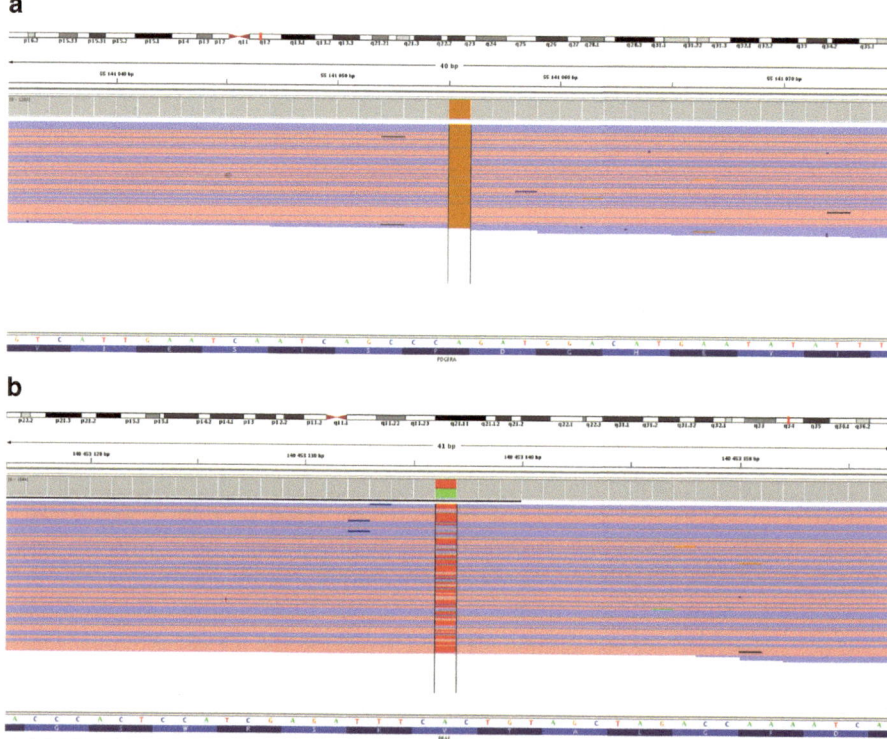

Fig. 6.12 Germline and somatic variants. (**a**) IGV screenshot of recurrent variant in PDFRA gene. (**b**) Example of somatic mutation *BRAF* V600E

A germline variant is a variation that an individual inherits from their parents. In a normal tissue, a SNV is expected to fall into one of the three bins: 0, 50, or 100 %, depending on whether it is heterozygous or homozygous. In case of common variants frequently observed in the population, the latter may be referred to as a single-nucleotide polymorphism (SNP). A somatic variant is a variation acquired by an individual which is not transmitted to the descendant. In oncology, a somatic variant refers to a mutation that occurs in a tumor. Their detection is indispensable to understand tumorigenesis and develop personalized therapies for patients (Fig. 6.12).

Distinct types of variations can occur and are classified according to their functional impact on the protein function:

- A *nonsense mutation* is a change in the DNA sequence which will produce a stop codon in the transcribed RNA and thus a truncated and/or nonfunctional protein.
- A *missense mutation* is a nonsynonymous change in the DNA, resulting in the change of an amino acid and thus in a nonfunctional or abnormal protein.
- A *neutral mutation* is a substitution of an amino acid that will not impact the protein function. Note that a neutral mutation usually refers to the use of a different but chemically similar amino acid, whereas a silent mutation will refer to a change in the DNA sequence that does not impact the nature of the amino acid.
- A *frameshift mutation* is caused by an insertion or a deletion which will change the reading frame of the translation resulting on a completely different protein.

The detection of short insertion and deletion (indels), germline, or somatic mutations usually requires distinct bioinformatics tools. Some variant callers are based on mathematical models to detect homozygous or heterozygous variants and are thus not suitable to detect very rare somatic mutations with a low frequency. Other bioinformatics solutions have been proposed to detect somatic mutations by comparing a pair of normal and tumoral samples, reporting the tumor-specific mutations.

Data Preprocessing

Previous works demonstrated that the Phred-like quality scores issued by the sequencing platforms may often deviate from the true error rate (Li et al. 2004). A couple of preprocessing steps have been proposed to improve the variant calling. These steps are independent from the calling itself and can be used before any variant caller. If they are thus not mandatory, they are usually advised to improve the sensibility and specificity of the variant calling (Van der Auwera et al. 2013).

The Genome Analysis ToolKit (GATK, McKenna et al. 2010) proposes to first calibrate the quality scores by treating every reference mismatch as indicative of sequencing error and by estimating the empirical quality score. Note that true polymorphisms are excluded from the process as they represent legitimate mismatches to the reference. Recalibrated quality scores are then estimated by adding to the raw quality scores the residual differences between empirical quality scores and the mismatch rates estimated from the raw quality scores. As an example, after alignment and filtering, a SAM file could contain only reported Q25 bases. However, it may be that these bases actually mismatch the reference at a 1 in 100 rate, so are actually Q20. The GATK recalibration score will correct the average quality inaccuracy by shifting from Q25 to Q20 but will also take into account the sequencing context, such as the fact that mismatches are more likely observed at the end of the reads or that some dinucleotides have often much lower qualities than others.

GATK also proposes a local realignment process to correct from misalignments around the indels. Indels are usually very difficult to align for a number of reasons:

(1) The penalty score of most alignment softwares is often much higher for the gap penalties than for the SNVs. Therefore, alignment softwares will preferentially allow SNVs than indels.
(2) The read mapping is performed independently for each read. It is therefore unlikely that all reads support the same mismatches pattern, especially for the reads starting/ending exactly at the beginning/end of the indels.
(3) Finally, a complicating issue is that short insertions and deletions often localized near-identical repetitive sequences which can create high rates of false positives. Therefore, it is often essential to consider haplotypes that include enough unique surrounding sequence to unambiguously evaluate evidence for the presence or absence of a deletion or insertion event with respect to the reference. The local realignment process will allow to realign reads with misalignments due to the indels into clean reads alignment supporting a consensus indel (Fig. 6.13).

Germline Variant Calling

The principle of germline variant detection is simple. At each position on the genome (or covered loci), the genotype is obtained by counting the number of occurrences of each nucleotide among the aligned reads. In case of homozygous

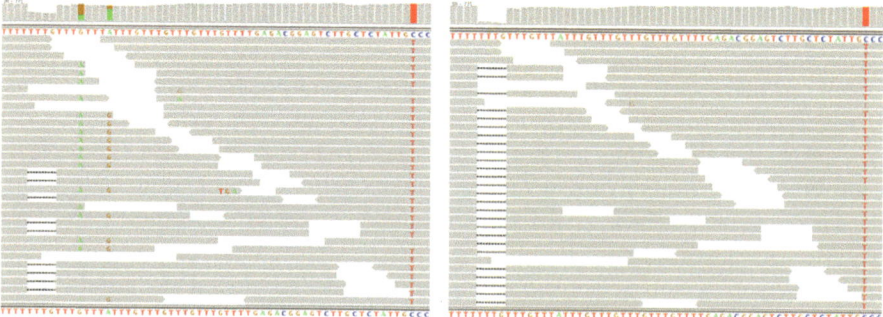

Fig. 6.13 Local realignment around indels. Example of local realignment process to correct from misalignments around the indels (GATK). On the *left*, the aligner preferentially allows SNVs instead of indels. On the *right*, the results of local realignment around indels

variants, all nucleotides should match the same allele, A or B. And in case of heterozygous variants, half of the nucleotide should match an A, when the other half should match a B. Many different softwares have been proposed to detect germline variants. The goal of these tools is to predict the likelihood of a variation for a given locus, based on the quality scores and allele counts of the aligned reads at that locus. Modern methods are mainly based on probabilistic programming and Bayesian modeling. One major advantage of the Bayesian framework is the use of prior information for an SNP at a given position such as allele frequencies and patterns of linkage disequilibrium. These prior probabilities can be derived from databases of known SNPs such as the dbSNP or from the calling of multiple individuals at the same time. The variant calling routines implemented in SAMtools and GATK both support the use of multiple samples calling. Briefly, it is assumed that one can compute the genotype likelihood $p\,(X|G)$, where G is a given genotype and X are the reads covering a given genomic position. Bayes' formula is used to calculate $p\,(G|X)$, which is the posterior probability of genotype G. The genotype with the highest posterior probability is usually chosen and used to compute a measure of confidence. The result is a variant, a genotype, and an associated measure of uncertainty (which is often described by a score), all of which have a concrete statistical interpretation.

Somatic Variant Calling

The detection of somatic variant is a critical step for cancer genome characterization and clinical genotyping. Working with a sufficient read depth is crucial to detect such event. If a read depth of 30X is usually enough to detect germline mutation in a normal tissue, at least 60X is advised for tumor sequencing. Detecting low-allelic-fraction SNVs in a sample is often important for early diagnosis, targeted therapy, and detection of residual tumors. In this context, targeted sequencing of a gene panel has been widely used to increase the variant detection sensitivity by achieving a much higher read depth (>500x), even on a benchtop sequencer. This strategy thus allows to detect rare variants on a panel of genes with a good accuracy.

Compared to the germline variant calling, additional factors usually affect the detection of somatic events:

- The contamination by the normal tissue leading to lower variant allele frequency
- The subclonal variants, which may occur in any fraction of the cells, meaning that the basal level of a heterozygous variant might be much lower than 50 %, depending on the tumor's clonality
- The copy number variants, neutral loss of heterozygosity, or ploidy changes, all of which leading to a shift of the expected variant fractions
- The nonnormal tissue, such as peritumoral sample use as control which can be contaminated by tumor cells

A first naive approach to detect somatic variant is to call the variants on a tumor sample and to screen the set of predicted SNVs against databases such as dbSNP (Sherry et al. 2001). The main limitation of this method is that there are around three millions of SNVs per individual. The first results from the 1 K Genome Project indicated that 10–50 % of these are novel events (Durbin et al. 2010). This suggests that possibly millions of SNVs in a single individual will be uncatalogued in polymorphism databases. These SNVs will be falsely identified as somatic mutations based on this strategy. To overcome this limitation, an accurate detection of somatic variants requires both the tumoral and the matched normal samples from the same individual. In general, these methods either perform the variant calling independently on both samples and then subtract both results or simultaneously analyze both samples using joint probability-based statistical approaches. As for germline variant calling, the somatic callers are usually based either on a Bayesian probabilistic or on a heuristic framework. In this context, instead of using a Bayesian framework and prior information to calculate genotype probabilities, variant calls are based on adjustable minimum thresholds for coverage, base quality, variant allele frequency, and statistical significance.

In general, agreement among different algorithms is relatively low, making the selection of candidate SNVs for further validation difficult (O'Rawe et al. 2013). This disagreement is likely partially due to different error models and prior assumptions underlying each algorithm. It is therefore advice to test and merge the results from multiple softwares.

Short Indel Detection

Short indels are a common and functionally important type of sequence polymorphism. However, the detection of these events from next-generation sequence data is challenging, and so far methods for identifying indels lag behind methods for calling SNVs in terms of sensitivity and specificity. Accurate detection of indels from short-read data is challenging for a number of reasons. First, compared with SNVs, indels occur at lower rates, which makes them more difficult to detect. Second, as previously discussed (see Sect. 6.2.2.5.3), reads arising from indel sequence are generally more difficult to map to the correct location in the genome. Therefore, using a local realignment method as proposed by the GATK suite allows to improve the reads mapping and detection accuracy. Two major paradigms are currently used for detecting short indels. The first one and most common approach is to align all of the input reads to the reference genome and to apply a detection method usually based on Bayesian probabilistic framework (Albers et al. 2011). The second paradigm consists of performing *de novo* assembly of the reads and to detect variations between the assembled contigs and the reference genome. More recently, Narzisi et al. proposed a microassembly approach using both reads mapping on a reference genome and de novo assembly. The main idea is to first use a standard mapping approach to distinguish well-mapped reads and reads that fail to fully align but are anchored on the genome. Those reads are then used to perform a microassembly in a local region (i.e., an exon) using a de Bruijn graph approach.

Variant Annotation

The detection of variants on exome-capture data generates a list of several thousand variants. One of the most challenging tasks is to filter and order these variants in order to pinpoint the driver mutations. Some bioinformatics tools such ANNOVAR (Wang et al. 2010), SNPEff (Cingolani et al. 2012), and Oncotator (Ramos et al. 2015) have been developed to annotate these variants. The input of these softwares is a Variant Calling Format (VCF) file which is the reference format to store the variants and annotation information.

The Human Genome Variation Society (HGVS) proposed a standard variant nomenclature, which should be used by researchers and diagnostic center in order to describe and classify the variants. The HGVS recommended nomenclature starts with a "*c.*" for variant in a coding region, "*r.*" for changes at the RNA level, and "*p.*" for the protein level. Details and examples about the HGVS nomenclature can be found in the http://www.hgvs.org/ website. Briefly, the most common changes are the following (see Fig. 6.5):

- *A nucleotide substitution* is represented by "*c.*" followed by the position of the substitution and the nucleotide change. For example, *c.76A > C* denotes that at nucleotide 76, an A is changed to a C. Substitution 5′ of the translation initiation codon and 3′ of the termination are, respectively, coded by the "*c.-*" and "*c.**" characters. Note that intronic variants can also be encoded using the "+" or "−" character. For example, *c.88 + 1G > T* denotes the G to T substitution at nucleotide +1 of an intron (in the coding DNA positioned between nucleotides 88 and 89) and *c.89-2A > C* denotes the A to C substitution at nucleotide −2 of an intron (starting from the nucleotide 89).
- *Amino acid substitutions are* encoded following the same model. For example, *p.Trp26Cys* refers to a change between tryptophan 26 to a cysteine. Note that a stop codon is encoded with the "*" character.
- *Insertions and deletion* are, respectively, designated by "*ins/del*" after the description of the nucleotides flanking the insertion/deletion site and followed by the inserted/deleted nucleotides. For example, *c.76_78delACT* denotes an ACT deletion from nucleotides 76–78 and *c.76_77insT* a T insertion between nucleotides 76 and 77 of the coding DNA reference sequence.
- *Amino acid insertion and deletion* are designated following the same nomenclature. Glutamine-8 (Gln, Q) deletion is therefore encoded as p.Gln8del. Note that frameshift changes are coded using the "fs" character. For example, *p.Arg97Hisfs*5* denotes a frame shifting change with arginine-97 as the first affected amino acid, changing into a histidine, and the new reading frame ending in a stop at position 5.

In addition, the list of detected variants can be annotated using many different external databases. Annotations usually include gene names, functional consequence, predictions of deleterious impact (PolyPhen), and cancer-specific annotations from resources such as COSMIC, Cancer Gene Census, Tumorscape, or dbSNP results.

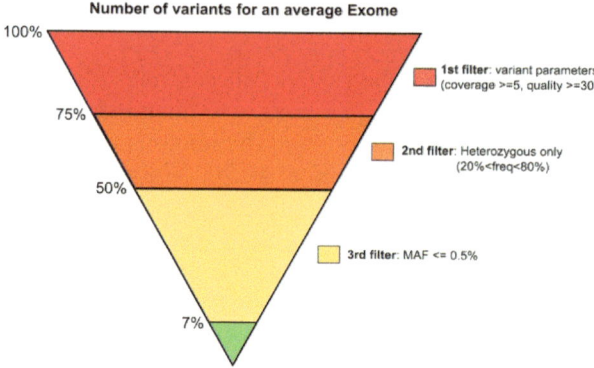

Fig. 6.14 Example of variant filtering. Different filters have to be applied to highlight causal mutation and discard noninformative variants. A first filter on variant quality allows to discard 25 % of variants. The second filter was applied to focus on heterozygous variants and the last one to keep only variants with a mean allele frequency lower than 0.5 % in control population

Variant Filtering

No matter how good the mutation caller is, there are going to be some false positives. It was recently shown that every sequencing technology as well as every variant caller will detect specific true variants. It is therefore crucial to filter out and order the list of variants. The exhaustive list of filters to apply usually depends on the biological context. A few common sources of false positives were already characterized as strand bias, homopolymer sequences, and reads on paralogous region of the genome and can be removed from the list of detected variants.

Figure 6.14 presents an example of filtering process used to highlight the driver mutations. Working with only high-quality reads, uniquely aligned on the genome with a *MAPQ* of at least 30, usually limits the false positives associated with sequencing or mapping errors. A true variant should be supported by a sufficient level of information, such as a minimum of 30× coverage and at least 5 distinct mutated reads. Variants that do not pass the quality filters of the softwares are also likely to be false positive. Finally, the environment of the variant can also be used. It is therefore recommended to remove variants from homopolymer or low complexity regions or with more than two other SNVs called within 10 bp. Sites passing these criteria are subjected to additional annotation filters. A screen against germline variants from dbSNP helps in discarding variants which match the position and allele of known noncancer dbSNP. Common polymorphisms found on more than 1 % of the ESP or 1000 Genomes Project population as well as recurrent, silent, and neutral variants can also be discarded. These variants do not present any therapeutic interest but are good internal controls to ensure the quality of the sequencing data. The Catalogue of Somatic Mutations in Cancer (COSMIC, http://cancer.sanger.ac.uk/cosmic) can be used to annotate the variants against known cancer mutations. It is however important to keep in mind that all these databases are far from perfect and have to be used with caution. For instance, the

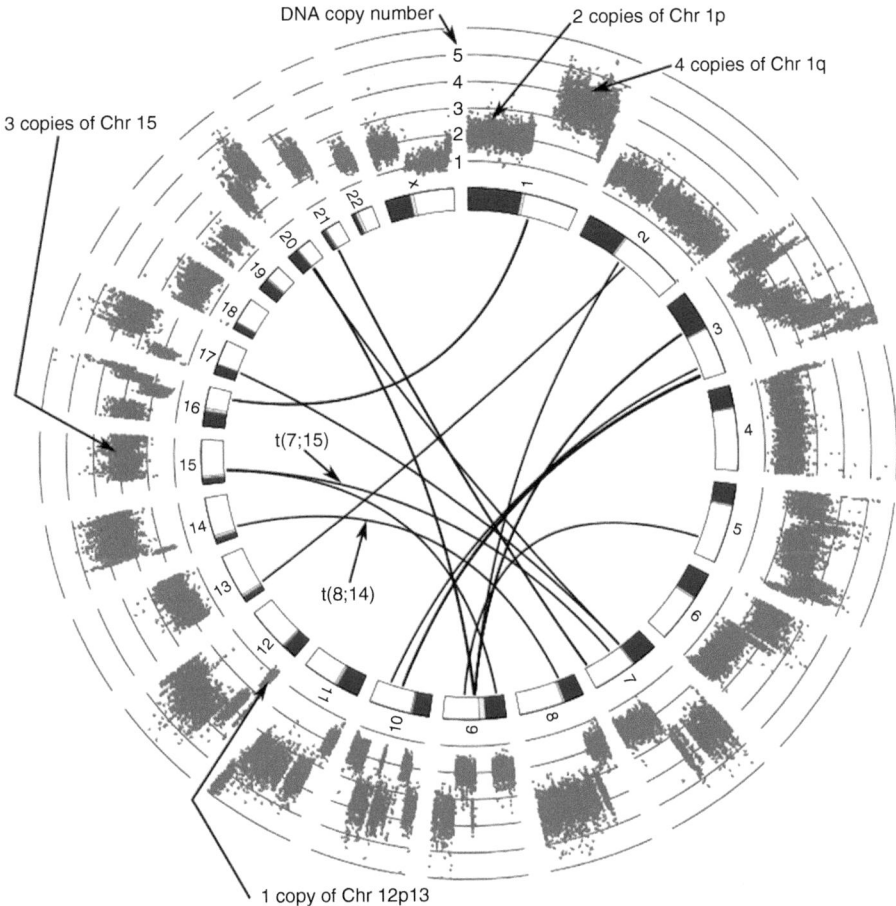

Fig. 6.15 Copy number and structural variants. Example of Circos view to summarize copy number variants and structural variants. Copy number changes of T47D cell line is represented as gain or loss. Interchromosomal translocations are represented by lines linking to two chromosomes

COSMIC database tends to become a reference today for cancer screening but is not exhaustive and contains a significant number of SNPs which are not true cancer driver mutations.

Structural and Copy Number Variation

The detection of germline or somatic variants remains today the main NGS-based clinical application. But other genomic variants can be detected using DNA sequencing approach. Recurrent chromosomal rearrangements are hallmarks of many cancers. Structural genomic rearrangements and copy number variations (CNVs) are usually associated with changes in gene expression (over-/down-expression) or can lead to chimera proteins through fusion genes.

Structural variants (SVs) can be identified using paired-end or mate-paired sequencing strategy (Fig. 6.15). Paired-end and mate-paired sequencing strategies mainly differ in the expected distance between the two mates (insert size) which is usually around 300 base pairs for paired-end data and up to 3 Kb for mate-paired data. It means that the probability of covering a breakpoint is higher with mate-paired strategy but that paired-end data can be very attractive to identify precise breakpoints location. The principle of bioinformatics solutions dedicated to SVs detection is to use the reads orientation and the insert size to detect and classify abnormal pairs (Zeitouni et al. 2010). A split reads approach can also be used in complement by some softwares.

CNVs can also be detected using sequencing data (Fig. 6.15). Bioinformatics solutions rely on the assumption that the depth of coverage is proportional to the number of DNA copies. Using a paired control sample is usually recommended in order to distinguish CNV from bias signal. However, some recent method can now estimate CNVs without control sample. Additional normalization procedure is thus required, such as a GC-content normalization (Boeva et al. 2011).

If whole-genome sequencing is therefore the method of choice to explore CNVs status of a tumor, its cost and the amount of data generated can be a limiting factor. For this reason, recent methods were proposed to explore CNVs using exome sequencing data (Tan et al. 2014). Of course, exome sequencing will not allow detecting rearrangements into intronic or intergenic regions, but it can be sufficient to detect amplified or lost genes within a tumor. Once again a control sample is highly recommended to estimate the noise coming from the capture protocol itself. Although the exome sequencing consists of in-depth sequencing of nearly all the coding exons, the amplicon sequencing technique aims at sequencing a limited number of genes at a lower cost. The genes included in a panel of amplicon sequencing are genes that are often altered in different cancer types (oncogenes or tumor suppressors) and for whose alterations targeted therapies have been established or are in clinical development. Detecting CNVs from target sequencing can therefore be very interesting for clinical purposes and is still open to discussion. Indeed, in terms of methodology, this question addresses new challenges of normalization and statistical confidence of the results. Detecting such events in amplicon sequencing data relies on the same main principle as exome or whole-genome sequencing, but the signal-to-noise ratio is more difficult to assess. Some methods start to emerge to detect amplified regions and require both control samples and a sufficient gene coverage.

6.2.2.6 Integrative Analysis and Reporting

The use of these new high-throughput technologies in clinics will generate a huge amount of information. In practice, there is a real need in defining a way to report to the clinician the results which can drive the clinical decision. This task is crucial and must be as complete and precise as possible but should also be summarized to allow a quick decision of the medical staff. Today, no report template was officially designed and shared to present the results of molecular profiles. We can however

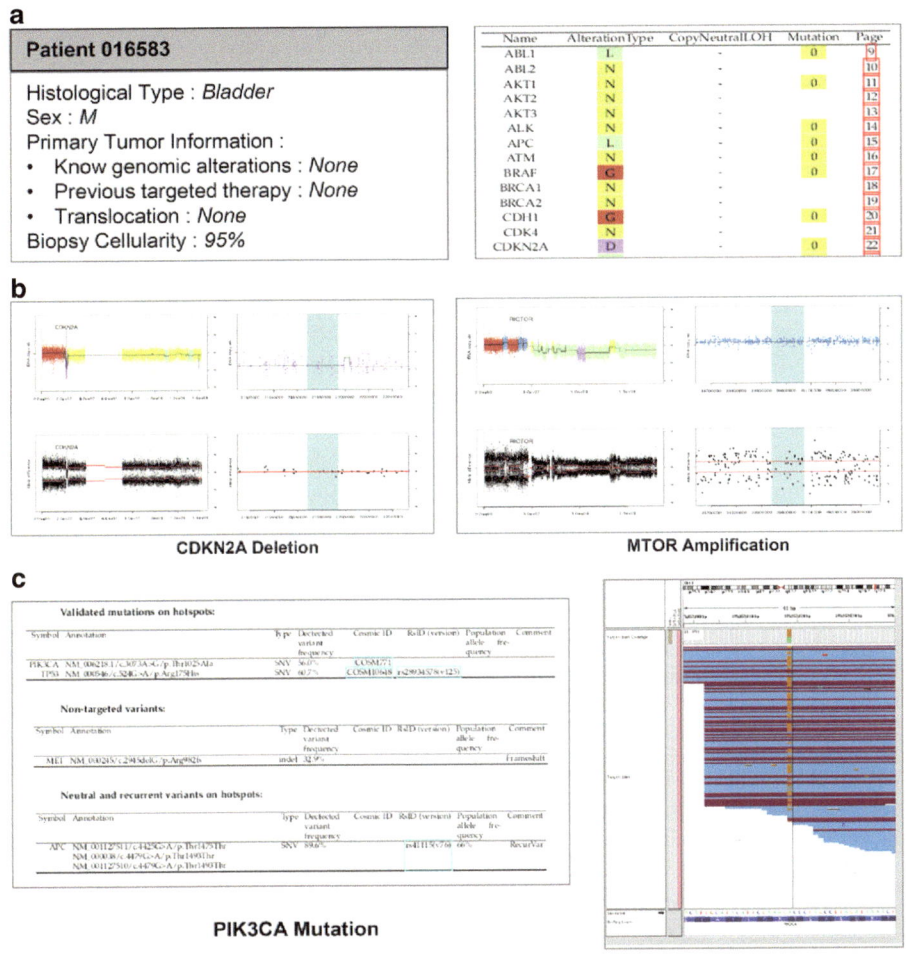

Fig. 6.16 Molecular profile report (SHIVA clinical trial). (**a**) Clinical and biological informations about the patient are reported to guide the therapeutic decision. DNA copy number and mutations statuses for all genes are reported in a table to provide a quick overview of the potential targets. (**b**) For each gene, detailed informations of their DNA gene copy number and loss of heterozygosity statuses are provided. (**c**) Mutations passing all the filters are reported as positives mutations. Nontargeted variants as well as recurrent variants are also reported. An IGV screenshot of the genomic region can help in validating the variant

illustrate the choices and the report used in the context of the SHIVA clinical trial (Fig. 6.16).

First, a report should present the clinical and biological information about the patient and the pathology (age, sex, histology, grade, treatment, etc.). Then, the molecular board will need to have access to the overall molecular profiles of the patient. This overview should help in detecting targetable alterations, validating the histology, and detecting potential technical issues. According to the context and the molecular profile, one way to summarize this information is to provide a table per gene, with the copy number alterations, LOH status, and mutations profiles.

One may think that this summarized information is enough to take a clinical decision. However, in practice, biologists and clinicians usually need more information about the genomic alteration. For instance, looking at the context around the alteration is usually very informative. Do we have other events in the same region? What is the exact size of the alteration? Is it focal or not? etc. Being able to have access to the annotation of the mutation is also required. What is the HGVS nomenclature of the variant? Is the mutation associated with a COSMIC ID? What is the context of the variant in homopolymer regions? etc.

Many of these informations can be automatically provided to the molecular board. In the context of the SHIVA trial and in addition to the summarized view per gene, clinicians and biologists can have access to a detailed description of each event with graphical views of the copy number profiles of each gene, as well as the list of mutations with detailed annotation. These additional data can be delivered as a technical report or accessible using an integrative information system.

6.2.3   From Research to Clinics

6.2.3.1   Development of Sustainable Bioinformatics Analysis Pipelines

As illustrated in the previous sections, the use of high-throughput technologies for precision medicine is unambiguously linked to the capacity of developing, maintaining, and using an adequate bioinformatics environment (Servant et al. 2014).

Maintaining an efficient bioinformatics workflow in a clinical context is today challenging because of the frequent updates of the computational solutions either installed on the sequencing machine or provided as stand-alone applications. These frequent updates are mainly due to the rapid evolution of the sequencing and microarray technologies but remain a major issue to ensure the operability of the bioinformatics pipelines and their reproducibility. As a consequence, any update requires that each bioinformatics pipeline was validated to ensure a high specificity and sensitivity. Any change in the data format or in the analysis methods can have critical consequences on the downstream analysis and results.

Moreover, many different methods are currently available to analyze NGS data, but no consensus or standard computational tools exist so far. For instance, detecting germline or somatic mutations can be achieved using different bioinformatics algorithms, tools, and filters. Choosing the most efficient algorithm is not an easy task, and a feasibility phase is mandatory to define which algorithms and parameters to apply for a dedicated question.

Several commercial solutions are available either with the sequencers themselves or as stand-alone applications. The use of such solution can be very attractive especially for laboratory without any bioinformatics support. However, their main limitation remains that these tools are usually presented as "black box" without any detail on the method or additional filters applied to deliver the final results. In addition, these solutions are usually not scalable and are not designed to follow the rapid evolution of kits or sequencing technology.

6.2.3.2 Sequencing the Genome and Beyond

Current NGS techniques expand from targeted sequencing based on a couple of genes to exome or whole-genome sequencing. The latter is today mainly used in cancer research and can be seen as the future of the clinical investigation. However, their use in routine clinical practice is much more difficult, mainly because the average depth of coverage is much lower than for targeted gene sequencing complicating mutation detection. However, these applications offer new ways to explore CNVs and SVs and can thus be used as an alternative to the current microarray technologies.

In addition, the current sequencing capabilities also offer new opportunities to develop gene/transcript expression and epigenomics biomarkers in clinic. For instance, the detection of *BRCA1*/BRCA2 isoforms and their quantification using RNAsequencing approach would be an interesting complementary approach to mutations screening (Houdayer et al. 2012). In the same way, epigenetics mechanisms such as DNA methylation, histone modifications, small noncoding regulatory RNAs, and nucleosome remodeling are also known to be involved in many biological processes and tumorigenesis. Alteration in epigenetic mechanisms can lead to somatic mutations, and somatic mutations in epigenetic regulators can lead to an altered epigenome (Timp and Feinberg 2013). If drug discovery in cancer epigenetics had been held back due to concern about specificity and toxicity, it remains an active field of investigation (see Dawson and Kouzarides, 2012, for a review).

These new fields also raise the question of combined therapies. The combination of targeted therapy with chemotherapy or with other targeted therapies is challenging because of increased toxicity.

Solutions include the use of lower doses of drugs which might not be relevant if the biologically active dose is not reached and the use of drugs in a sequential manner although the relevance of this approach still needs to be demonstrated. For instance, it is likely that the combination of standard chemotherapy together with drugs against mutated proteins and epigenetics drugs offers synergistic benefits and therefore increases therapeutic efficacy. Integrative analysis considering together genome, proteome, and epigenome is a major challenge to explore the complexity of the disease and to identify new therapeutic targets.

References

Albers CA, Lunter G, MacArthur DG et al (2011) Dindel: accurate indel calls from short-read data. Genome Res 21(6):961–973. doi:10.1101/gr.112326.110.arXiv:10040887v1

Athey BD, Braxenthaler M, Haas M et al (2013) tranSMART: an open source, and community-driven informatics, and data sharing platform for clinical, and translational research. AMIA Jt Summits Transl Sci Proc 2013:6–8

Boeva V, Zinovyev A, Bleakley K et al (2011) Control-free calling of copy number alterations in deep-sequencing data using GC-content normalization. Bioinformatics 27(2):268–269

Burrows M, Wheeler DJ (1994) A block sorting lossless data compression algorithm. Technical report 124. Digital Equipment Corporation, Palo Alto

Canuel V, Rance B, Avillach P et al (2014) Translational research platforms integrating clinical, and omics data: a review of publicly available solutions. Brief Bioinformat. doi:10.1093/bib/bbu006

Cerami E, Gao J, Dogrusoz U et al (2012) The cBio cancer genomics portal: an open platform for exploring multidimensional cancer genomics data. Cancer Discov 2:401–404. doi:10.1158/2159-8290.CD-12-0095

Cingolani P, Platts A, Wang-le L et al (2012) A program for annotating and predicting the effects of single nucleotide polymorphisms, SnpEff: SNPs in the genome of Drosophila melanogaster strain w1118; iso-2; iso-3. Fly 6(2):80–92

Dawson MA, Kouzarides T (2012) Cancer epigenetics: from mechanism to therapy. Cell 150(1):12–27. doi:10.1016/j.cell.2012.06.013

Downing GJ, Boyle SN, Brinner KM et al (2009) Information management to enable personalized medicine: stakeholder roles in building clinical decision support. BMC Med Inform Decis Mak 9:44. doi:10.1186/1472-6947-9-44

Durbin RM, Abecasis GR, Altshuler RM et al (2010) A map of human genome variation from population-scale sequencing. Nature 467(7319):1061–1073

Fernald GH, Capriotti E, Daneshjou R et al (2011) Bioinformatics challenges for personalized medicine. Bioinformatics 27:1741–1748. doi:10.1093/bioinformatics/btr295

Houdayer C, Caux-Moncoutier V, Krieger S et al (2012) Guidelines for splicing analysis in molecular diagnosis derived from a set of 327 combined in silico/in vitro studies on BRCA1 and BRCA2 variants. Hum Mutat 33(8):1228–1238. doi:10.1002/humu.22101

Hupé P, Stransky N, Thiery J-P, Radvanyi F, Barillot E (2004) Analysis of array CGH: data: from signal ratio to gain and loss of DNA regions. Bioinformatics 20:3413–3422. doi:10.1093/bioinformatics/bth418

Langmead B, Salzberg SL (2012) Fast gapped-read alignment with bowtie 2. Nat Methods 9(4):357–359. doi:10.1038/nmeth.1923

Langmead B, Trapnell C, Pop M et al (2009) Ultrafast and memory-efficient alignment of short DNA sequences to the human genome. Genome Biol 10(3):R25. doi:10.1186/gb-2009-10-3-r25

Li M, Nordborg M, Li LM (2004) Adjust quality scores from alignment and improve sequencing accuracy. Nucleic Acids Res 32(17):5183–5191

Li H, Handsaker B, Wysoker A et al (2009) The Sequence Alignment/Map format and SAMtools. Bioinformatics 25(16):2078–2079. doi:10.1093/bioinformatics/btp352

Madhavan S, Gusev Y, Harris MA (2011) G-CODE: enabling systems medicine through innovative informatics. Genome Biol 12(Suppl 1):P38. doi:10.1186/gb-2011-12-s1-p38

Marco-Sola S, Sammeth M, Guigo R et al (2012) The GEM mapper: fast, accurate and versatile alignment by filtration. Nat Method 9:1185–1188. doi:10.1038/nmeth.2221

McKenna A, Hanna M, Banks E et al (2010) The Genome Analysis Toolkit: A MapReduce framework for analyzing next-generation DNA sequencing data. Genome Res 20:1297–1303

O'Rawe J, Jiang T, Sun G et al (2013) Low concordance of multiple variant-calling pipelines: practical implications for exome and genome sequencing. Genome Med 5:28. doi:10.1186/gm432

Popova T, Manié E, Stoppa-Lyonnet D, Rigaill G, Barillot E, Stern MH (2009) Genome Alteration Print (GAP): a tool to visualize and mine complex cancer genomic profiles obtained by SNP arrays. Genome Biol 10:R128. doi:10.1186/gb-2009-10-11-r128

Ramos AH, Lichtenstein L, Gupta M et al (2015) Oncotator: cancer variant annotation tool. Hum Mutat 36:E2423–E2429, http://dx.doi.org/10.1002/humu.22771

Rigaill, G. (2010). Pruned dynamic programming for optimal multiple change-point detection. ArXiv e-prints, (May):9

Servant N, Roméjon J, Gestraud P et al (2014) Bioinformatics for precision medicine in oncology: principles and application to the SHIVA clinical trial. Front Genet 5:152. doi:10.3389/fgene.2014.00152

Sherry ST, Ward MH, Kholodov M, Baker J, Phan L, Smigielski EM, Sirotkin K (2001) dbSNP: the NCBI database of genetic variation. Nucleic Acids Res 29(1):308–311

Simon R, Roychowdhury S (2013) Implementing personalized cancer genomics in clinical trials. Nat Rev Drug Discov 12:358–369. doi:10.1038/nrd3979

Tan R, Wang Y, Kleinstein SE et al (2014) An evaluation of copy number variation detection tools from whole-exome sequencing data. Hum Mutat 35(7):899–907. doi:10.1002/humu.22537

Timp W, Feinberg AP (2013) Cancer as a dysregulated epigenome allowing cellular growth advantage at the expense of the host. Nat Rev Cancer 13:497–510. doi:10.1038/nrc3486

Van der Auwera GA, Carneiro M, Hartl C et al (2013) From FastQ data to high-confidence variant calls: the Genome Analysis Toolkit best practices pipeline. Curr Protoc Bioinformatics 43:11.10.1–11.10.33

Veltman JA, Cuppen E, Vrijenhoek T (2013) Challenges for implementing next-generation sequencing-based genome diagnostics: it's also the people, not just the machines. Personal Med 10:473–484. doi:10.2217/pme.13.41

Wang K, Li M, Hakonarson H (2010) ANNOVAR: functional annotation of genetic variants from high-throughput sequencing data. Nucleic Acids Res 38, e164. doi:10.1093/nar/gkq603

Zeitouni B, Boeva V, Janoueix-Lerosey I et al (2010) SVDetect: a tool to identify genomic structural variations from paired-end and mate-pair sequencing data. Bioinformatics 26:1895–1896. doi:10.1093/bioinformatics/btq293

Chapter 7
Assessment of Biomarkers' Predictive Value of Efficacy

Etienne Rouleau, Céline Callens, Gaëlle Pierron, and Ivan Bièche

7.1 Introduction

The tumor molecular screening faces different challenges. There is a large diversity of alterations from point mutations to chromosomal alterations at the genomic levels (please refer to Chap. 3). The level of the allelic frequency in the sample can vary from zero to 100 % and the mutation signal can be hampered by the normal tissue contamination. These alterations mean different methods of detection. High-throughput sequencing and whole genome copy number detection with techniques such as CGH array can bring sensitive information for tumor analysis.

Cancer is caused by alterations in the control and activity of genes that in turn regulate cell growth and differentiation, leading to abnormal cell proliferation. Cancer-related genes include two classes of genes, which have opposite effects: Tumor-suppressor genes (TSG) normally repress cell growth, while oncogenes normally stimulate cell growth. In this context, the genetic alterations in cancer involve abnormal activation of oncogenes (gain of function) or inactivation of TSG (loss of function). Oncogenes' gain-of-function alterations act dominantly, i.e., only one of the two alleles is sufficient for activation and cancer induction. On the other hand, TSG loss of function needs the alteration of two alleles to induce cancer. The identification of the two alterations can be difficult with some variants which can have dominant effect. Activations of oncogenes usually result from (1) activating point

E. Rouleau, PharmD, PhD (✉) • C. Callens, PharmD, PhD • G. Pierron, PhD
Department of Genetics, Institut Curie, Paris, France
e-mail: etienne.rouleau@curie.fr; celine.callens@curie.fr; gaelle.pierron@curie.fr

I. Bièche, PharmD, PhD
Department of Genetics, Institut Curie, Paris, France

Department of Genetics, EA7331, University of Paris-Descartes, Paris, France
e-mail: ivan.bieche@curie.fr

© Springer International Publishing Switzerland 2015
C. Le Tourneau, M. Kamal (eds.), *Pan-cancer Integrative Molecular Portrait Towards a New Paradigm in Precision Medicine*,
DOI 10.1007/978-3-319-22189-2_7

mutations; (2) localized reduplication (DNA amplification) that includes the ónco-gene, leading to overexpression of the encoded oncoprotein; and (3) chromosomal translocation resulting in a change of the promoter and abnormal expression of the oncogene in question or a fusion transcript encoding for a chimeric protein. Inactivation of TSG usually results from (1) inactivating point mutations, (2) homo-zygous or heterozygous deletions of DNA segments that include the TSG, and (3) epigenetic inactivation of the promoter.

Once the variants are identified on a gene with sequencing and/or copy number assessment, the second step is the interpretation of the variant in question. The nature of the variant is different depending on the nature of the gene, i.e., oncogene or TSG. Indeed, a stop codon is probably not of interest in any oncogenes and a missense variant has a lower probability to be causative in a TSG. If for the onco-genes, such as *KRAS* gene, the range of mutations is limited to few hotspots, the situation is different for suppressor genes such as *TP53* gene in which the number of mutation possibilities is unlimited although some regions concentrate most of the mutations. With high-throughput sequencing, the number of the detected vari-ants is consequently more important pinpointing the key step of variant interpreta-tion. Consequently, it is very important to use the terminology of "variant" at this first level of interpretation. The role of the biologist is then to classify variant as "driver" alteration, which can be investigated as a biomarker. Drivers can be designed as "mutation" and have often functional impact on the protein. He can also classify other variants as a "passenger" alteration, which is a random conse-quence of the genomic instability (Hanahan and Weinberg 2011; Vogelstein et al. 2013). Some variants are also single-nucleotide variants (SNP) (>1 %) or rare vari-ants (<1 %) present in the general population, for which no impact is described on the protein.

The goal of this chapter is to present the steps undergone by the biologist to ensure the functional interpretation of a specific variant, which can become a marker of prediction in personalized medicine decision.

The production of sequences and the identification of genomic variants are the bottleneck of the molecular labs. Today, the main challenge becomes the interpreta-tion of a large set of genomic variants to make it usable for clinical decision and in enough confidence to ensure the best therapeutic decision. Initially, a companion biomarker – a gene and a list of mutations – was identified for a drug in clinical tri-als. There were only few hotspot mutations with clear impact on the prediction of treatment's response. Molecular platforms were stimulated to screen only those hotspots. High-throughput sequencing extends the genetic screening with far more genes, in which entire coding sequences are sequenced. Therefore, the number of variants discovered is increasing independently from any clinical evidence of their utility. The interpretation of the activation of some variants is sometimes only based on functional cellular data and without the same level of evidence than the initial mutations identified in the pivotal clinical trial. There is then an inference of the clinical impact. The assessment of molecular results is becoming increasingly complex.

In this chapter, the value of biomarker will be discussed with the evidence collected through clinical, *in vitro*, and basic research. The distinction between activating/inactivating impact and predictive impact will be stressed. Afterward, interpretation guidelines will be discussed to help the reader enter the molecular expertise for biomarkers' interpretation (Fig. 7.1).

7.2 Technical Validation of the Variant

The first role of the molecular biologist is to technically analyze the molecular result to insure the interpretation of the detected variant. This assessment is done with the help of bioinformaticians who have developed script processes to present the list of variants and exclude any false positive with a proper selection of filters.

In fact, the technology by itself can lead to large numbers of false-positive, especially in the case of variant detections with low level of mutated alleles. Many protocols try to identify variants suggesting identification of minor subpopulations at low level. The low detection threshold will increase the risk of false positives.

Biologists need to know the technological noise background, which is dependent on the method used. With next-generation (NGS) sequencing, the error rate of the Illumina technology is estimated to be <0.4 % with MiSeq or HiSeq technologies (Quail et al. 2012). The error rate with Ion Torrent sequencing has been estimated to

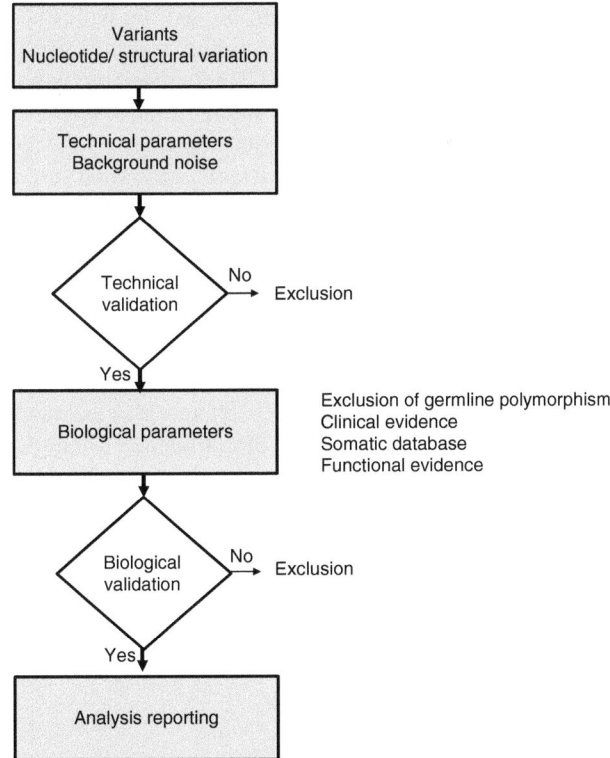

Fig. 7.1 Variant validation steps

2 % (Quail et al. 2012). The recurrence of those errors is one of the ways to identify them. Some variants are located at the beginning or the end of reads and then can be trimmed in the analysis.

False positive can also be generated by the quality of the DNA and sample preparation. In the formalin-fixed paraffin-embedded (FFPE) specimens, noise can result from both low quantity of DNA and cytosine deamination to uracil (Do and Dobrovic 2012). Those artifacts are nonreproducible within replicates. Several strategies can be proposed from qualification of the DNA before any enrichments or dedicated treatment either during the extraction or the amplification.

For the NGS, the risk of false negative is related to the material and the kit design as well as the bioinformatics' process. One of the main challenges in tumor analysis is the range of allelic frequencies. As the goal of the somatic sequencing analysis is also to be able to detect low level of mutation, the threshold of the allelic frequency is often under 5 % and close to the background noise. The Sanger sequencing cannot be used in that case to validate a mutation detected by NGS since its sensitivity is limited to 10 %. The cellularity should also be considered to interpret the results as a low level of tumor cell percentage in the sample will lead to a reduction of the sensitivity. The technical validation process is also important and the biologist should be ensured that the approach is able to detect most of the recurrent somatic alterations. The use of internal and external controls is one of the means to validate the bioinformatics' process and avoid any false negative due to changes in the process.

False negatives can finally result from a bad coverage of the analyzed genomic region. The in silico analysis of the bed file with the covered region and with the CGHa coverage and oligonucleotide position is also an important step to validate the covered region. Indeed, for TSG, there are rarely hotspots of mutations and a full coverage is needed to correctly interpret the result.

All those points are crucial to be addressed by the biologist before any interpretation. It is important to validate the design and be sure that the results are reproducible with the use of well-selected controls.

7.3 Biological Interpretation

Once the presence of a molecular alteration is technically confirmed, the biological interpretation will add a level of confidence to consider the identified variants as actionable. The main goal of the interpretation is to predict the potential functional impact and to validate mutations as "driver" and exclude any "passenger" or "polymorphism." Finally, the variants will often remain as "unclassified" since no evidence can be identified for any classification.

7.3.1 Nucleotide Variation

The genomic analysis of tumor samples leads to the identification of variants which can be identified in all cells of the patient, germline variants, or which are only identified in the tumoral sample and then identified as somatic variants. In most the tumor characterizations, the sequencing analysis, mainly with targeted sequencing, is done without any information on the germline variants of the patient. The analysis of the germline DNA is a key step for reducing false positives (Jones et al. 2015). A different strategy using database analysis is then necessary to exclude the germline variants in a list of identified alterations. The recurrence of a variant in many samples can be a clue to identify a polymorphism. However, the recurrence of a variant in a series of tumors is not an argument in favor of a polymorphism as some mutations as in the gene *KRAS* or *PIK3CA* are recurrent.

7.3.1.1 Exclusion of Polymorphism

The germline variant database will help distinguish a polymorphism from a somatic mutation. The two databases frequently used are the 1000 genome and the Exome Variant Server (EVS). The 1000 genome gathers the information from 2500 unidentified people through the world with exome analysis. The EVS gathers the information from 5400 patients which have noncancer disease (http://evs.gs.washington.edu/EVS/). A threshold of 0.1 % can be used to distinguish SNP from somatic mutations (<0.1 %).

The database dbSNP is not recommended to directly classify variants. This database gathers many variants, which have been identified independently of the systematic screening. In this database, the curation of the variant is not strict enough as some somatic mutations have been included with reference number (rs). The current version is the build 142. The selection of SNPs with a minor allele frequency (MAF) of 1 % or greater can be a reasonable threshold for excluding germline variants common in the general population.

Mendelian disease can also help for the classification of variants. In fact, if the variant is related to a Mendelian disease, it should not be a polymorphism. The *TP53* mutations are related to Li–Fraumeni syndrome which can help to classify variants. Identically, the mutations of the von Hippel–Lindau tumor-suppressor gene are specific for the clear-cell histologic subtype of renal cell carcinoma related to von Hippel–Lindau syndrome. Several locus specific databases exist as UMD database for the gene *BRCA1* and *BRCA2*. The ClinVar database (http://www.ncbi.nlm.nih.gov/clinvar/) is an attempt to gather all the information about germline variants throughout all the genes.

7.3.2 Somatic Mutation Database

Most driver mutations are recurrent in several tumoral processes and should be identified into the tumor databases. The Catalogue of Somatic Mutations in Cancer (COSMIC) contains a comprehensive catalog of over 136,000 somatic coding mutations in over 500,000 tumor samples. The limit of COSMIC is the fact that the statistics are based on different technical approaches of screenings with mainly hotspot analysis for mutations' detection.

The whole exome sequencing (WES) of thousands of tumors as compared to germline exome sequencing to exclude SNPs has now been performed both by individual groups and through collective efforts such as the International Cancer Genome Consortium (ICGC) and the Cancer Genome Atlas (TCGA). The tumor bioportal give the access to the exome from different tumors (www.tumorportal.org or www.cbioportal.org). The list of somatic mutated genes looks finally limited in number when crossing all the TCGA from 12 major cancer types (Kandoth et al. 2013). The somatic variant database can help to identify some driver mutations, yet they can contain "passenger" variants. Consequently, the identification of recurrence of the variant in those databases could be a positive argument in favor of driver impact of the mutation.

7.3.3 Functional Evidence

Once the variant is not considered as a polymorphism or constitutional variant, other impacts need to be assessed. First of all, a variant can have impact on the splicing, which can cause the deletion of several nucleotides of one or several exons in the RNA transcript leading to functional impact. Secondly, a missense variant can lead to a functional impact by switching the amino acid. To identify those effects, one can assess the predictive value of biomarker for the splicing and for the protein function. For the splicing, the MaxENtScan is the best tool available and proves to be the most performant (Houdayer et al. 2012). Splicing can lead to oncogenic effect as the *MET* skipping of exon 14 in lung cancer which activates the tyrosine kinase activity (Seo et al. 2012). The splicing information is also very useful for predicting an inactivation of the suppressor genes.

On the other hand, the *SIFT* and PolyPhen algorithms help to understand the effect of the mutation on the amino acid. The validation of this system has been tested in Mendelian disease (Valdmanis et al. 2009). The validity is less obvious for oncogenes as the prediction is only about loss of function, whereas in oncogene, a functional gain is needed.

For oncogenes, the protein expertise is very useful. The alignment interspecies can be proposed and are integrated in *SIFT* and PolyPhen data bases. The alignment between proteins with the same function can be also a way to bring some information.

That is the case of the tyrosine kinase receptors (*EGFR, MET, ERBB2*, etc.). The alignment of those proteins will help to have a good knowledge of the most sensitive region which could have an impact on the activation of the protein and more specifically their kinase domain.

That is why the functional assays are the best solution to explore and definitely give an interpretation of the functional impact of the variants. The case of *PIK3CA* gene is very interesting since several mutations have been reported but the functional impact is very different for each mutation (Gymnopoulos et al. 2007). Currently, without enough rapid testing, the functional informations in the literature on variants are very useful for the classification. One would speculate that prospective *in vivo* assays might be possible to be performed in the furure to contribute to the interpretation of rare variants.

7.3.4   Copy Number Variants

The most common approach to identity copy number variants is the CGH-array (CGHa) approach or SNP-array approach. Identically to the NGS analysis, several steps are needed to reduce the list of alterations to targetable variants. On the CGHa, some background noise can be interpreted as amplification or deletion. The validation of the quality of the profile is the first important steps. Secondly, a minimal number of oligonucleotides implied in the alteration (i.e., more than 3) are the parameter used to exclude such false positive.

The existence of copy number polymorphisms should also be examined to be excluded. The comparative hybridization of the germline DNA is really the best way to exclude germline copy number variants. If no germline DNAs are available, the use of database can be the solution. The database of copy number polymorphisms is the Database of Genomic Variants (http://projects.tcag.ca/variation/). This database gathered copy number variants (CNVs), insertions/deletions (InDels), inversions, and inversion breakpoints annotated observed in healthy individuals and involving segments of DNA that are larger than 1000 bp. Insertions/deletions of 50 bp or larger are also included.

The size can be a good way to identify those variants for oncogenic alteration. The number of copies of a specific oncogene that reflects its potential amplification needs to be interpreted by taking into account tumor cellularity and ploidy. Only focal amplifications with ≥6 copies and less than 10 Mb in size could be considered relevant. In fact, a short amplification region size increases the probability of the implication of the gene included in the region. The level of the amplification intensity will really depend on the percentage of normal tissue. The best example remains the *ERBB2* amplification in breast cancer, which is still very focal. On the other hand, large amplifications or gains (>10 Mb) should not be considered unless validated by another technique such as IHC. In fact, there are often many genes in a large region which reduce the chance of identification of any driver.

Some chromosomal alterations can indirectly activate the pathway of the drug activity. That is why it is also pertinent to position any deletion/amplification into the protein pathway to identify any indirect implication. For instance, an amplification of the PDPK1 gene can lead to propose an anti-mTor therapy as this protein is in the *PIK3CA*-mTOR pathway. The publicly available database Kegg can be a good starting point to identify the protein interactions (http://www.genome.jp/kegg/pathway.html) and ease this interpretation. The exploitation of copy number alteration will certainly anticipate the exploitation of whole exome analysis.

Finally, for the deletion of TSG, the size seems less important especially if there is a deleterious mutation or a LOH reported in the second allele. For TSG, the expression of the protein needs to be abolished either with double mutation, combination of mutation and deletion, or a double homozygous deletion. The deletion or loss of heterozygosity can be very useful in the interpretation of variants in TSG. In fact for TSG, only loss-of-function homozygous mutations are considered deleterious and hemizygous mutations where the second allele is lost (somatic uniparental isodisomy). The loss of both alleles can also be interpreted as a full suppression of the function of the TSG. In those cases, the size of the alteration is not necessary a good indication, but the combination of deleterious mutation and loss of heterozygosity can be useful to indicate a role of the TSG in the tumor process.

7.3.5 Cross Validation

The integration of results from different techniques and different molecular levels is a key step for the interpretation of genomic variants. Many programs try to integrate DNA, RNA, mutation, and chromosomal alteration in the analysis. For instance, any deletion of *PTEN* can be confirmed with the IHC of the protein. On the other hand, an amplification or deletion could be validated with the RNA expression or with FISH assays. In the context of cancer-suppressor genes, the interpretation of the loss of the second allele can be done with CGH array to confirm the biallellic inactivation of the TSG.

7.3.6 Clinical Evidence

Unfortunately, the clinical evidence to associate a mutation to a drug response is very low for most of the mutations identified. Currently, the only clinical data available are for the gene as *KIT* (Heinrich et al. 2003) or *KRAS* (Karapetis et al. 2008; Van Cutsem et al. 2011) in solid tumor. They are more and more documented through clinical trial and also Mendelian disease. To classify a variant, there is more and more need for extrapolation.

7.3.7 Clinical Report

When all those selection processes are finalized, the variant can be reported. One can propose the following protocol. Variants should be described by the nomenclature HGVS with genomic reference NM and a clear statement of the value of the variant needs to be reported.

The following classes of variants can be accepted depending on the level of evidence: actionable variant, no theranostic evidence but with an activator potential effect (oncogene) or an inactivating potential effect (suppressor gene), no functional evidence with favorable data modeling, potentially neutral variant, and neutral polymorphism. The University of North Carolina at Chapel Hill (UNC) proposes a two-tier classification. First tier is variants with a well-known druggable alteration for which there is no ambiguity in the clinical use such as some *KRAS* mutations in colorectal cancer or some *EGFR* mutations in lung cancer. The second tier covers the genetic alterations of potential clinical significance: 2A for which targeted drug is commercially available, 2B with clinical trials, 2C considered druggable, and finally 2D with prognostic value are reported as well (Neil Hayes et al. 2015). The remaining variants are considered as of unknown significance and need to be discussed in a multidisciplinary group.

The role for the biologist is then to provide obvious information about those variations. However, it is now better to report all the variants except potentially neutral/neutral as the clinical evidence and clinical trial shift rapidly. Finally, the molecular staff will integrate those data to decide the treatment with this information. Some tumor will have several actionable molecular alterations. The goal is clearly to give a hierarchy to the information. The example of the tumor with both a *STK11* nonsense mutation and an *ERBB2* mutant which is also found as a resistance mutation in *EGFR* will lead to the preference on the *STK11* nonsense mutation, which is more directly interpretable (personal information). It is clear also that an activating impact does not mean predictive impact.

The implication of a molecular biology board (MBB) in the decision is then relevant as more and more targets are identified in the biological report. The utilization of algorithms in the decision process will also help for the prioritization, especially in clinical trials.

7.4 Challenges

The extension of the targeted genes from a short list to the whole exome will be the progression of the technical coverage. Additional information will be integrated from RNA-seq (Roychowdhury et al. 2011). This extension will consequently increase the complexity in the analysis of information. However, other next challenges will be the integration of several data in the clinical decision process from the complexity of the tumoral process, the tumor heterogeneity, and ctDNA.

First of all, the NGS of DNA is not sufficient to grasp all the complexity of the tumoral process (Pennington et al. 2014). The experience shows, for instance, the importance to integrate also CGHa information and certainly the RNA-seq will be the next step. The assessment of the immune system in the cancer therapy is becoming a new point of inclusion. Several applications can be proposed from vaccination strategy to immune checkpoint blockade. The expression of PD-L1 have a high negative predictive value for the efficacy of anti-PD-L1 therapy (Topalian et al. 2012) but other markers need to be added. Recently, the instability of microsatellite will certainly be included in the decision of treatment with immunotherapy (Xiao and Freeman 2015). Identically, the *BRCA1/2* alterations identified in ovarian cancer are divided into mutations for both genes and also methylation of *BRCA1* promoter {Ctation}. The impact of those methylations needs to be assessed in the antiPARP1 therapeutic strategies. Additional analysis will include exome for neoantigen identification, RNA sequencing, proteomics, polychromatic flow cytometry, methylome, etc. One of the main challenges will be to integrate all these results in one report for the clinician to orient therapeutic decision. Most of the significance of those markers remains unknown.

As the technique is more and more sensitive, subclonal alterations can be identified in tumor. The characterization of the tumor is usually performed on a single sample. The heterogeneity of tumor has been now well characterized (Gerlinger et al. 2012). The knowledge of this subclonal variant could help to assess the prognosis depending on mutations which can confer resistance. The increase of the limit of detection with the NGS will provide this information. However, a low level of *KRAS* could be enough not to decide to treat the patient (Laurent-Puig et al. 2015). Of note, the interpretation of potential resistance biomarker needs to be considered differently when compared to sensitivity biomarkers when it comes to low-frequency molecular alterations. Iterative sampling should better help to identify this relevant heterogeneity. The question remains "when does the biologist need to report this information?"

Finally, circulating tumoral DNA (ctDNA) will certainly provide valuable information for the patient management and help to estimate the tumor heterogeneity. This information will strongly modify the way to work with tumoral samples. NGS should be one of the techniques to detect those circulating mutations (Lebofsky et al. 2015). This certainly should be integrated as supplementary information. Many elements need to be assessed concerning the real capacity of ctDNA to bring additional information as to subclonal variants in case of resistance. More and more trials now accept ctDNA results. The anti-*EGFR* treatment can now be prescribed with this sole information in adenocarcinoma of lung cancer. The next steps will be the follow-up of ctDNA and the detection of additonal molecular information. The evidence produced looks promising for the prediction of clinical outcomes (Mok et al. 2015). Some CNV can also be detected as the *HER2* amplification in gastric cancer (Shoda et al. 2014). Finally, the application of exome will open the possibility to integrate both point mutation and chromosomal alteration (Murtaza et al. 2013). The current limitation of all those technique is the sensitivity which is close to 70 % and still need to be assessed toward the tumoral tissue information.

7.5   Conclusions

Variant classifications will help the decision for the choice of precision medicine that is mostly adapted to the tumor alteration. The decision in the classification should be based both on external information from databases and more and more on internal information as copy number variants, RNA level, DNA methylation, etc.

The expression can also be altered with different mechanisms leading to either variation into the RNA transcription or directly variation into the protein level.

Those variations are not systematically related to a genomic alteration and can be the result of epigenetic modifications.

The integration in real time of all those informations in a unique report will be certainly the next challenge for clinical decision and MBB. It is now relevant to follow the impact of this decision to improve the information on variants and their clinical implication. That is why the best framework of those decisions should be in a clinical trial and in a molecular staff assessing precisely the clinical benefit. Several challenges will surge as the increase of variants and altered molecular pathways to be interpreted but also the integration of other assays into the report.

References

Do H, Dobrovic A (2012) Dramatic reduction of sequence artefacts from DNA isolated from formalin-fixed cancer biopsies by treatment with uracil- DNA glycosylase. Oncotarget 3:546–558

Gerlinger M, Rowan AJ, Horswell S et al (2012) Intratumor heterogeneity and branched evolution revealed by multiregion sequencing. N Engl J Med 366:883–892

Hanahan D, Weinberg RA (2011) Hallmarks of cancer: the next generation. Cell 144:646–674

Heinrich MC, Corless CL, Demetri GD et al (2003) Kinase mutations and imatinib response in patients with metastatic gastrointestinal stromal tumor. J Clin Oncol Off J Am Soc Clin Oncol 21:4342–4349

Houdayer C, Caux-Moncoutier V, Krieger S et al (2012) Guidelines for splicing analysis in molecular diagnosis derived from a set of 327 combined in silico/in vitro studies on *BRCA1* and BRCA2 variants. Hum Mutat 33:1228–1238

Jones S, Anagnostou V, Lytle K et al (2015) Personalized genomic analyses for cancer mutation discovery and interpretation. Sci Transl Med 7:283ra53

Kandoth C, McLellan MD, Vandin F et al (2013) Mutational landscape and significance across 12 major cancer types. Nature 502:333–339

Karapetis CS, Khambata-Ford S, Jonker DJ et al (2008) K-ras mutations and benefit from cetuximab in advanced colorectal cancer. N Engl J Med 359:1757–1765

Laurent-Puig P, Pekin D, Normand C et al (2015) Clinical relevance of *KRAS*-mutated subclones detected with picodroplet digital PCR in advanced colorectal cancer treated with anti-*EGFR* therapy. Clin Cancer Res Off J Am Assoc Cancer Res 21:1087–1097

Lebofsky R, Decraene C, Bernard V et al (2015) Circulating tumor DNA as a non-invasive substitute to metastasis biopsy for tumor genotyping and personalized medicine in a prospective trial across all tumor types. Mol Oncol 9:783–790

Mok TSK, Wu YL, Soo Lee J et al (2015) Detection and dynamic changes of *EGFR* mutations from circulating tumor DNA as a predictor of survival outcomes in NSCLC patients treated with first-line intercalated erlotinib and chemotherapy. Clin Cancer Res Off J Am Assoc Cancer Res

Murtaza M, Dawson SJ, Tsui DWY et al (2013) Non-invasive analysis of acquired resistance to cancer therapy by sequencing of plasma DNA. Nature 497:108–112

Quail MA, Smith M, Coupland P et al (2012) A tale of three next generation sequencing platforms: comparison of Ion Torrent, Pacific Biosciences and Illumina MiSeq sequencers. BMC Genomics 13:341

Roychowdhury S, Iyer MK, Robinson DR et al (2011) Personalized oncology through integrative high-throughput sequencing: a pilot study. Sci Transl Med 3:111ra121

Seo JS, Ju YS, Lee WC et al (2012) The transcriptional landscape and mutational profile of lung adenocarcinoma. Genome Res 22:2109–2119

Shoda K, Masuda K, Ichikawa D et al (2014) *HER2* amplification detected in the circulating DNA of patients with gastric cancer: a retrospective pilot study. Gastric Cancer Off J Int Gastric Cancer Assoc Jpn Gastric Cancer Assoc

Topalian SL, Hodi FS, Brahmer JR et al (2012) Safety, activity, and immune correlates of anti-PD-1 antibody in cancer. N Engl J Med 366:2443–2454

Valdmanis PN, Verlaan DJ, Rouleau GA (2009) The proportion of mutations predicted to have a deleterious effect differs between gain and loss of function genes in neurodegenerative disease. Hum Mutat 30:E481–E489

Van Cutsem E, Kohne CH, Lang I et al (2011) Cetuximab plus irinotecan, fluorouracil, and leucovorin as first-line treatment for metastatic colorectal cancer: updated analysis of overall survival according to tumor *KRAS* and *BRAF* mutation status. J Clin Oncol Off J Am Soc Clin Oncol 29:2011–2019

Vogelstein B, Papadopoulos N, Velculescu VE et al (2013) Cancer genome landscapes. Science 339:1546–1558

Xiao Y, Freeman GJ (2015) The microsatellite instable subset of colorectal cancer is a particularly good candidate for checkpoint blockade immunotherapy. Cancer Discov 5:16–18

Chapter 8
Designs for Evaluating Precision Medicine Trials

Xavier Paoletti, Bernard Asselain, and Christophe Le Tourneau

8.1 Introduction

During the last two decades, the majority of new agents have been designed to target molecular alterations involved in carcinogenesis. Most of these agents are expected to produce antitumor activity only in the presence of the matching molecular alteration or companion biomarker. The objective of treating patients based on the molecular profile of their tumor is claimed by most of the sponsors and investigators.

This vast field of research covers various objectives such as the identification of the target population that may benefit from a treatment, the validation of a prognostic or predictive biomarker to treat patients, and the investigation of complex algorithms to select the adequate treatment among a set of several agents in a single or in multiple diseases. For each of these questions, one or several designs have been proposed, implemented, or discussed. In this chapter, we focus on the issue of designing trials with multiple tumor types and/or multiple treatments to assess the added value of a predefined algorithm. Readers interested in the statistical designs

X. Paoletti, PhD (✉)
Biostatistics and Epidemiology Department, INSERM U1018,
Gustave Roussy Cancer Campus, 114 rue Ed Vaillant,
94805 Villejuif, France
e-mail: xavier.paoletti@gustaveroussy.fr

B. Asselain, MD, PhD
Biostatistics Department, INSERM U900, Institut Curie, Paris, France
e-mail: bernard.asselain@curie.fr

C. Le Tourneau, MD, PhD
Department of Medical Oncology, Institut Curie, Saint-Cloud, Paris, France

EA7285, Versailles-Saint-Quentin-en-Yvelines University, Versailles, France
e-mail: christophe.letourneau@curie.fr

© Springer International Publishing Switzerland 2015
C. Le Tourneau, M. Kamal (eds.), *Pan-cancer Integrative Molecular Portrait Towards a New Paradigm in Precision Medicine*,
DOI 10.1007/978-3-319-22189-2_8

tailored for the investigation of biomarkers for a single treatment in a disease are referred to several high-quality contributions that make a comprehensive review of the various approaches (Buyse and Michiels 2013; Sargent et al. 2005).

To date, molecularly targeted agents (MTAs) have been assessed according to tumor location and histology. Investigations in other tumor types are then pursued on a case-by-case basis. For instance, trastuzumab first got approval in *HER2* amplified breast cancer before it was investigated in advanced/metastatic stomach cancers overexpressing *HER2* (Bang et al. 2010). However, this approach is rapidly limited by the sample sizes required for clinical trials: the combination of the (low) prevalence of some alterations as well as some specific tumor types transforms several subgroups into rare diseases. The sequential development of a MTA in multiple tumor types with the same molecular abnormality is thus unrealistic in most cases. Therefore, there is strong interest in the possibility to investigate several tumors with common biological characteristics in the same trial.

The general question of whether personalized medicine based on the molecular profiling of the tumor of cancer patients improves their outcome has arisen. In a prospective cohort study, Von Hoff and colleagues concluded to the benefit of selecting treatment for refractory cancer based solely on the tumor biology (Von Hoff et al. 2010). In a comparative non randomized trial, Tsimberidou and colleagues reported that in patients with at least one druggable molecular alteration identified in their tumor, matched MTA compared with treatment without matching was associated with a higher objective response rate, longer progression-free survival (PFS), and longer survival (Tsimberidou et al. 2014). However, the lack of randomization *versus* standard of care in these studies did not allow drawing robust conclusions (Buyse et al. 2011). The aim of these studies is no longer to investigate a unique biomarker but to study whether an algorithm is predictive of the response to treatment, which raises numerous challenges.

To illustrate the various methodological questions we need to address to set up a trial in this context, we use the SHIVA trial as a running example. It was designed to evaluate whether tumor biology is a more important driver for treating cancer patients than tumor location and histology. This randomized trial compared molecular targeted wtherapy approved at the time of the trial (outside of their approved indications) based on metastasis molecular profiling *versus* chemotherapy (or best supportive care) at investigators' choice in patients with any kind of cancer refractory to standard of care. The intervention evaluated in this trial can be described as a complex algorithm that determines the association of a treatment with a putative adequate target.

It is important to remind that the preliminary step before engaging in such scientific question is to assess the validity of the measure of the marker of activity (McShane et al. 2013). It must be shown to have all characteristics of diagnostic tests, which includes the reproducibility of the assay, the metronomic quality of the measures, and a high sensitivity and specificity. Many assays remain experimental, and, if used, one should be certain that the technique will not be modified during the course of the trial, which would considerably limit the interpretation of the final results. In the following, we will assume that this is available, even if in many situations, we might doubt of the validity of the theranostic marker.

In the following, we recall the fundamental difference between prognostic and predictive factors of response to treatment, and we emphasize the necessity of randomized trials to evaluate the predictive accuracy of molecular-based algorithms. We then introduce the rationale for the design, the choice of endpoints, the type of conclusions we can expect, and the specificities due to this type of clinical question. We review the main limits. In particular, we explore the power of randomized trials in case only part of the algorithm would be efficient, that is if only some MTAs actually work in the presence of the selected target while others do not. Finally, we present alternative designs and discuss their main features.

8.2 Prognostic and Predictive Factors

Prognostic and predictive factors of response to treatment are commonly confused. A prognostic factor is associated with the outcome (typically survival, PFS, response) and the natural history of a disease for a given population. For instance, patients with breast cancers that do not overexpress estrogen receptors (ER- tumors) have less good prognosis than women with ER+ tumors. ERBB2-amplified breast cancer tumors are associated with shorter overall survival or time to relapse. This association is not modified when the patient is treated with conventional chemotherapy (taxanes, for instance). On the contrary, predictive factors of response to treatment modify the treatment effect. In other words, predictive factors interact with the treatment effect. While a simple association measure characterizes prognostic factors, an interaction test and interaction measures are requested to determine predictive factors of response to treatment. The main consequence from a design point of view is that a prognostic factor can be identified on a single-arm cohort, but a predictive factor must be drawn from a comparative trial. This is illustrated in Fig. 8.1 taken from Paoletti et al. (2011). Predictive markers can be seen either as a variation of the treatment effect according to the marker value (first row of the panel) or as a variation of the prognosis in markers positive and negative patients according to the treatment arm (second row of the panel). This latter visualization highlights the fact that if only treated patients are studied, one may erroneously conclude to the absence of the marker's impact. Many predictive factors are also prognostic factors such as *HER2* with trastuzumab or estrogen receptors status with hormonal therapies. Only comparative trials enable to identify predictive factors of response to treatment.

8.3 Randomized Design of the SHIVA Trial

The primary objective of the SHIVA trial was to compare the efficacy in terms of PFS of molecularly targeted therapy based on molecular profiling *versus* conventional therapy as selected by the investigator in patients with solid tumors refractory to standard treatments. The concept appeared particularly attractive for less

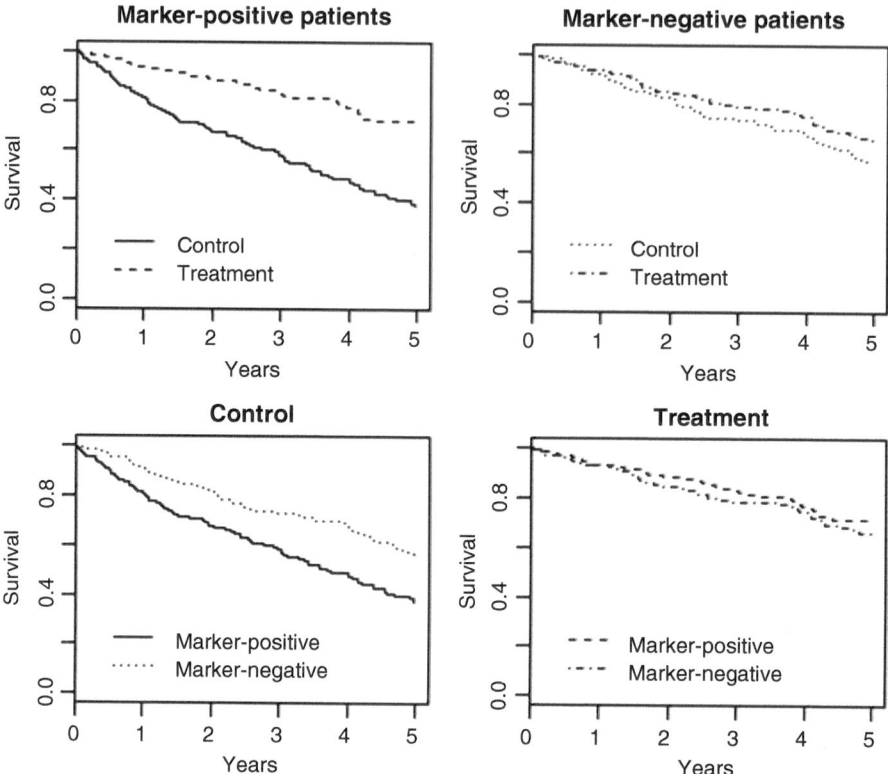

Fig. 8.1 Illustration of predictive factors of response to treatment. The upper panel gives typical survival obtained after treatment and after control in biomarkers positive (*left*) and biomarker nega- tive (*right*) patients. The lower panel presents the same data in a different way as survival curves are given for each biomarker category in the treatment arm (*left*) and in the control arm (*right*)

common or rare tumor types for which dedicated randomized trials of MTAs are usually not carried out (Le Tourneau et al. 2010). This supported the idea to include all solid tumor types that can be evaluated for efficacy using the same criteria. A very large set of MTAs is on the market or under development, with various levels of evidence of activity depending on the stage of development. We decided to use only approved drugs (that can be assumed to have demonstrated clinical benefit in some tumor types) in order to control for this source of heterogeneity.

8.3.1 Flowchart

The flowchart of the study is provided in Fig. 8.2. The SHIVA trial included an observation cohort study as well as a randomized trial. In brief, the molecular pro- file of a patient tumor was performed on a mandatory biopsy/resection of a metas- tasis and analyzed by a molecular biology board (MBB) composed of biologists,

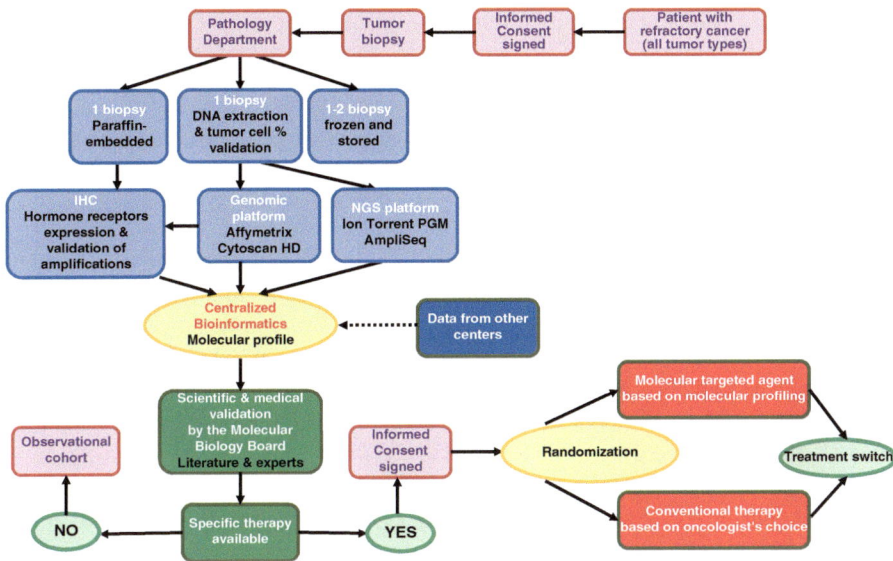

Fig. 8.2 Flowchart of the SHIVA trial

physicians, and bioinformaticians. If one or several molecular alterations were identified, the molecular biology board applied a predefined algorithm to select the best MTA. Patients were then randomized between receiving the selected MTA and receiving a conventional treatment according to the investigators choice (that is based on tumor type, histopathological characteristics, etc.). The investigator and the patient were blinded to the molecular profile (Le Tourneau et al. 2014). A cross-over was allowed at disease progression for patients in both treatment arms (patients who received conventional chemotherapy are proposed the MTA and vice versa).

8.3.2 Endpoints

Progression-free survival was defined as the delay between randomization and progression according to RECIST 1.1 (Eisenhauer et al. 2009) or death, whatever the cause. Secondary efficacy objectives were to investigate the tumor growth according to the treatment arm, to explore the possible variation in treatment effect according to the altered pathway (interaction test), and to compare the tumor growth obtained with the MTA and the standard treatments for patients who crossed over. Tumor growth was defined quantitatively as the sum of the size of the targeted lesions identified using RECIST 1.1 standardized by the delay between measurements. This endpoint, conceptually appealing, raises several practical issues: new lesions and clinical progressions are not part of the quantitative measures, which may entail conflicting evaluations compared to standard criteria. Furthermore, patients with early progression or death without CT scan measurements are excluded. Alternatively, joint modeling of both radiological and clinical outcomes can be envisaged, but statistical analyses are then challenging.

8.3.3 Heterogeneity in Patients' Prognosis

It is well known that prognosis differs depending on the tumor type, although patients with the same cancer in terms of location and histology might also display different prognosis (Le Tourneau et al. 2012). In order to control for this heterogeneity, randomization was stratified according to the signaling pathway relevant for the choice of the MTA and the patient prognosis based on the two categories of the Royal Marsden Hospital (RMH) score for oncology phase I trials (Olmos et al. 2012). Although molecular alterations may be prognostic for PFS, it was not possible to stratify the design for all possible molecular alterations. Three main signaling pathways have been arbitrarily identified: (1) the hormone receptors pathway, (2) the PI3K/AKT/mTOR pathway, and (3) the MAP kinase pathway. Therefore, combining the two levels of prognosis from the RMH score with the three molecular pathways, the randomization and the planned primary analysis were stratified on six strata. Last, quotas were introduced so that no more than 20 % of the randomized patients had the same tumor type.

8.3.4 Sample Size Calculation

The population of interest included various tumor types and various number of previous lines of treatment, similar to the population enrolled in phase I trials. The expected PFS of this population in the control arm could be derived from the one reported in phase I clinical trials of cytotoxic agents that have been eventually approved: 6-month PFS in this patient population was around 15 % (Horstmann et al. 2002). Under the hypothesis that doubling the 6-month PFS rate from 15 to 30 % was clinically relevant (i.e., HR = 0.63), a total of 142 events was required to detect a statistically significant difference in PFS between the randomized arms with a type I error of 5 % and a power of 80 % in a bilateral setting. To observe these events after an accrual time of 18 months and a minimum individual follow-up of 6 months, about 200 patients were needed to be randomized onto this trial.

8.4 Design Specificities Relating to the Use of High-Throughput Technologies

The evaluation of a complex intervention such as the algorithm to select the MTA raises specific issues that not only impact the design but also the statistical analysis and the final interpretation. First, this complex intervention combines two aspects: the treatment effect and the choice of the putative matching target. Therefore, the resulting efficacy can be related to either of the two, and the final interpretation is the evaluation of the whole strategy compared to another strategy (physician choice) which uses different treatments and a different modality to select the treatment. Second, several sources of variability related to the complexity of the intervention may contribute to the final results of the experiment. Eleven different targeted treatments have been administered based on 22 targets characterized by several dozen molecular alterations. A fundamental assumption behind the design is that the intervention has similar effects (or absence of effects) in all six strata, whatever the allocated treatment and whatever the molecular alteration used to select the treatment. This is the homogeneity assumption. In case the algorithm is only partly efficient, the power of the study is impacted. The magnitude of the impact is investigated in the following section. Third, as in any scientific experiment, the algorithm to select patients must be duly described, reproducible, and applicable to all participants. Defining the treatment algorithm was challenging as the knowledge regarding the biology of the tumors and the high-throughput platforms evolves quickly with time, and initial biological assumptions might become outdated. Platforms used the same protocol throughout the trial. Likewise, all bioinformatics analyses had to be centralized and applied to all patients regardless of recruitment center. No modification of the bioinformatics workflows was accepted during the project. Finally, all patients enrolled in the trial were analyzed in the same way. This is crucial as any research must be self-explanatory and reproducible. A treatment algorithm that would rely only on understated experts' opinion would not be applicable outside of the center, and conclusions would not be applicable and generalizable to other samples. This is a key condition to be able to scientifically evaluate the intervention.

8.4.1 Strengths of Randomized Designs

The various aspects of the design were carefully thought to answer the primary objective, limit the bias, and maximize the power with constrained resources.

8.4.1.1 Randomization

As introduced in Sect. 8.3, a randomized clinical trial is mandatory to evaluate the added value of omic-based classifiers to guide patients' treatment compared to standard approaches. Although the tumor biology, the mechanisms of drug resistance, and the role of the tumor environment are known to be crucial to accurately predict patient outcomes, they remain largely unknown, making it necessary to have a comparator. Furthermore, the prognosis of the highly selected patients (those whose tumors have a set of predefined molecular alterations) enrolled in such trials is not well known. Likewise, only an intent-to-treat analysis that makes full use of the randomization is appropriate. However, as shown in the next section, this is necessary, but this may not be sufficient to provide a clear picture of the benefit of the complex intervention.

8.4.1.2 Blinded Design

Blinding to the molecular profile is a crucial component to evaluate the benefit of the intervention (Boutron et al. 2006). The expectations of the physicians and of the patients in omic-based algorithms to select MTAs are high; there is a risk of bias in the follow-up as well as in the measure and interpretation of the primary outcome that are likely to favor the intervention arm. Ideally, a double-blind trial should be designed, which is delicate when several formulations, schedules, and agents are tested in the same trial.

8.4.1.3 Crossover

Crossover was allowed to patients at disease progression. Patients initially randomized in the intervention group may then receive conventional chemotherapy based on their tumor type, and patients in the control arm may receive the MTA matching the molecular alteration identified on the biopsy performed at inclusion, provided all eligibility criteria were still fulfilled at the time of progression. This gives a unique opportunity to compare both therapeutic strategies in the same patients using each patient as his/her own control. The randomization between the two arms of treatment can also be seen as a randomization between the two sequences of treatment, fulfilling one requirement of crossover designs. The statistical power of this analysis is theoretically higher than the one comparing the treatment efficacy between the two groups as it enables control for the various sources of patients related heterogeneity such as the natural history of the disease (the tumor location and histology), the history of previous treatments, etc., if the time to progression (TTP) for the two consecutive treatments are correlated (Buyse et al. 2011). Furthermore, in this planned crossover, all tumor evaluations are performed using the same criteria, the same set of target lesions identified prospectively. This gives a better and more robust assessment of the two consecutive TTP compared to retrospective assessment. However, in the likely event where a large fraction of patients cannot receive both arms (i.e., no crossover) due to clinical deterioration, for instance, the conclusions may be biased. Accordingly, the primary analysis should rely on the first period only. The main drawback of allowing crossover is to make any analysis of the overall survival meaningless.

8.4.1.4 Tumor Diversity

In clinical trials opened to all tumor types, distribution of disease depends strongly on the prevalence of the various cancers and the specific expertise of the participating centers. Yet, less common tumor types with frequent molecular abnormalities could benefit from the approach. To limit the risk that most patients have the same tumor type, which might preclude the generality of the results, heterogeneity in the tumor type can be increased by design. Setting up quotas for tumor types avoids overrepresentation of more frequent tumor types such as breast, lung, or colorectal cancers. Differences between the treatment arms would then be unlikely related to a given tumor type. This would reinforce the interest of developing new treatments based on biology first, possibly across multiple diseases. In summary, randomized designs allow for comparing two complex strategies on a valid endpoint while controlling for numerous confounding factors. A statistically significant difference between the two arms would be appropriately interpreted as the superiority of treating patients with MTAs based on molecular alterations and a predefined treatment algorithm compared to the conventional approach based on tumor location and histology. In other words, do we perform better than what we usually do for these patients?

8.4.2 Limitations of the Selected Design

The complexity of the question raised by such programs induces numerous limits to any statistical design. One may try to reduce the risk of biases or of inconclusive trial; this is however often not possible to avoid them totally.

8.4.2.1 Interpretation

An important question that will not be addressed in this type of trial is the independent effect of the algorithm. The design will not enable to disentangle the treatment effect from the algorithm effect. If a given MTA is active irrespective of the measure of the target (that is of the algorithm), we would draw the same conclusions as if the treatment worked due to the adequate selection of the patients.

The US national cancer institute sponsored M-PACT trial (NCT01827384) has been designed to specifically address the question of the added value of the algorithm regardless of the treatment effects. M-PACT focuses on four MTAs. Patients whose tumor expresses molecular alterations are randomized between the MTA matching the detected molecular alteration *versus* one of three other nonmatching therapy arms. In the latter case, the MTA is selected by the investigator blinded to the molecular profile. Only the added value of the algorithm is studied. Conversely, the control arm used in the M-PACT trial does not correspond to any standard of care, and the trial will not be able to conclude whether the global strategy is superior to the usual practice. Both types of trials are therefore quite complementary.

8.4.2.2 Population Heterogeneity

If randomization guarantees that the two groups of patients have comparable characteristics and the same overall prognosis, heterogeneity may dilute the expected benefit if the intervention effect is somehow modified by patients' characteristics. Heterogeneity impacts any clinical research, but several sources of potential heterogeneity across patients are specific for (or more likely with) this kind of trials of limited sample sizes: the location and histology of the tumor, the molecular alterations, the assays used to identify the molecular alterations, and the diversity of

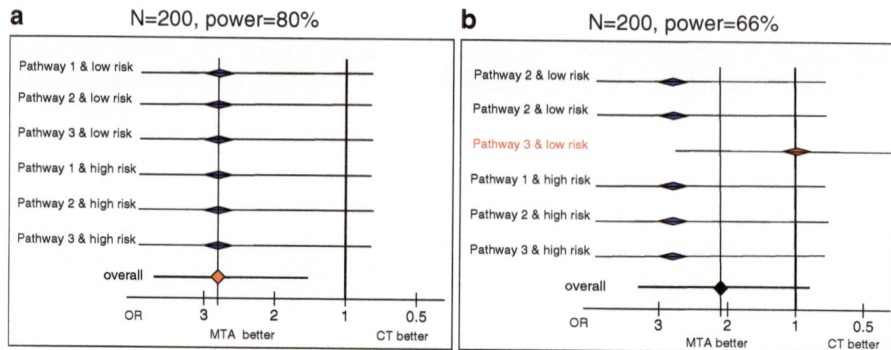

Fig. 8.3 Illustration of the loss of power if only part of the heterogeneity predicts the effect of treatment. Point estimates and 95 % confidence intervals (*horizontal lines*) are provided. (**a**) Homogeneous benefit of the targeted treatment selected based on molecular alterations in all strata; (**b**) benefit of the targeted treatment selected based on molecular alterations in all but one stratum. *OR* stands for odds ration; *MTA* for molecular targeted treatments; *CT* for chemotherapy; *N* gives the total sample size

treatments under study may impact the treatment effect. Stratification of the randomization and of the analysis on the RMH prognostic score and on the signaling pathway is an efficient mean to control heterogeneity in the prognosis of these various groups, assuming no interaction between the strata and the treatment effect (i.e. if the algorithm is relevant for all pathways as discussed in the following paragraph). It was impossible to stratify on the numerous tumor types. On the contrary, as noted in the previous section, we tried to increase the diversity of the tumor types to be able to draw conclusions that would be broadly applicable. This source of heterogeneity is intrinsic to the question addressed by the SHIVA trial, and we tried to build on it while controlling for the other identified sources of heterogeneity.

8.4.2.3 Treatment Effect Heterogeneity and Power

Beyond the expected heterogeneity in the population prognosis, there is a risk of heterogeneity in the effect of the MTA selected based on the molecular alteration. In other words, the algorithm to select the right treatment would be efficient for some molecular alterations (or equivalently for some treatments) and not for the others. For instance, in the SHIVA trial suppose that the treatment selected in case of an alteration on the PI3K/AKT/mTOR pathway is not active in this subset of patients, this would reduce the power of the primary analysis. Our ability to detect a 50 % reduction in the rate of progression or death at 6 months would be lower than the planned 80 %. This is illustrated by the forest plots in Fig. 8.3. Each line represents the MTA effect in a different stratum. For simplicity, PFS at 6 month is treated as a binary variable as if no patient was censored before a minimal follow-up at 6 months; the treatment effect is quantified by odds-rati (OR). In panel A, we have homogeneity of the treatment effect across all strata: whatever the signaling pathway and the prognostic group, the PFS rate is increased by 50 %. Conversely, in

Table 8.1 Power of the randomized comparative trial to detect an overall increase in the progression-free survival rate at 6 months from 15 to 30 % in case of heterogeneity assuming balanced prevalence of all six strata groups

Number of strata with MTA better	Power for the comparative test (%)	Power for heterogeneity test
6	80	–
5	66	25
4	49	36
3	32	38
2	17	34

In strata with no treatment effect, we assumed the same rate of progression at 6 months. Homogeneity is tested using Woolf's test

panel B, no treatment effect is observed in one of the strata, and the overall power of the primary analysis is reduced from 80 to 66 %.

The magnitude of the power loss depends on the number of strata where the MTA is not active, as shown in Table 8.1. The size of each stratum is also directly related to the power (results not shown). Homogeneity tests (or interaction tests) are part of the statistical analysis plan in order to detect this pattern of results. However, interaction tests are notoriously underpowered as shown in Table 8.1, and a strong heterogeneity may remain statistically undetected at the 5 % level.

8.4.2.4 Endpoints

The primary endpoint to evaluate treatment benefit in advanced disease is the PFS for many trials. As secondary endpoint, the quantitative measure of the tumor growth is analyzed (Le Tourneau et al. 2012). This endpoint has been increasingly investigated in recent years due to the potential increased information carried in continuous outcomes (Litière et al. 2014). In particular, an improved ability to detect interactions between the treatment effect and baseline characteristics such as the signaling pathway is expected. However, recent works have demonstrated that none of the endpoints based on the tumor growth proposed to date were a good surrogate of the patients survival (An et al. 2013), and this is not clear whether a treatment effect measured on the tumor growth would be strongly predictive of a treatment effect on the PFS. Furthermore, the best way to combine information from tumor growth and the occurrence of new lesions or clinical symptoms is still an area of research. This endpoint may help to provide a better understanding of some aspects of the data, but it could not be used as a primary endpoint instead of PFS.

8.4.3 Alternative Designs for Multi-tumors or Multidrugs Trials

Comparative designs play a central role to evaluate predictive markers of response to treatment. Noncomparative studies that were performed in some tumor types, such as the SAFIR 01 in breast cancers, gave impressive results on the feasibility and the possibility to match patients to drugs that might target identified molecular abnormalities, but they do not enable to validate predictive markers (including algorithms) of response to treatment (André et al. 2014) in absence of comparator. Randomization has numerous advantages detailed in previous sections. However, several variations have been explored to address the questions of the sample size that may be quite large due to the ratio between the number of patients to screen and the number of randomized patients as well as the issue of heterogeneity in the treatment effect.

8.4.3.1 Comparative Nonrandomized Designs

Patient as Their Own Controls

Several trials have proposed to use the patient as his or her own control (Rodon et al. 2015; Hollebecque et al. 2014). In the pilot study by von Hoff introduced in Sect. 8.2, the TTP obtained after the treatment based on molecular alteration is compared to the TTP of the previous line of treatment. For instance, assume that a patient failed two lines of treatment for metastatic disease before entering into the trial; one would compare the TTP of the third line with the one of the second line. Under the hypothesis that the natural history of cancer follows an exponential tumor growth (Ribba et al. 2014), one expects that the TTP of each line of treatment should be shorter and shorter. Therefore, the ratio of TTP can be categorized in a success/failure result based on some threshold; a ratio below 0.75 has often been selected. This underlying hypothesis can be expressed statistically as the existence of a strong correlation between two consecutive lines of treatment. The stronger the correlation is, the more powerful the statistical tests are as this approach controls for the intrapatient sources of variability. Few data have investigated this correlation that is probably dependent upon the tumor type. For instance, strong correlation has been reported in GIST tumors treated with two successive doses of imatinib (Zalcberg et al. 2005), but low correlations has been measured in colorectal trials (Tournigand et al. 2004). Furthermore, this endpoint has some strong limitations that include:

- The assessment of the TTP at the previous line of treatment that is commonly done retrospectively, which implies different evaluation criteria (RECIST is not systematically used in clinical practice to define progression), different means of investigation, or different target lesions.
- The use of TTP rather than PFS as an endpoint as death cannot be included in the first evaluation.
- Conclusions may be biased as we cannot control for the period effect as in a standard crossover design (where the sequence of treatments is randomized).

A single-arm trial is then designed; a cohort of patients is treated based on molecular abnormalities until progression; the time to progression is compared to the one obtained at the previous line. Following works by Mick et al. (2000), sample size calculation to detect a ratio between paired TTP can be computed if the expected correlation is known. Let us denote this ratio $TTPR = TTP_2/TTP_1$ where TTP_2 is the outcome of the investigational strategy. Under the null hypothesis, TTPR > γ where gamma is some value describing the expected ratio if the investigational strategy is inefficient. Von Hoff proposed to take $\gamma = 1.33$. Suppose that most of the observations are not censored and that we can use a paired sign rank test for the sample size calculation. In case of censored observation, alternative Gehan-Wilcoxon test Jung (1999) could be used. For the ith patient, let r_i be equal to

$$+1 \quad \text{if} \quad TTP_2 > TTP_1 * \alpha \tag{8.1}$$

$$-1 \quad \text{if} \quad TTP_2 \, TTP_1 * \gamma \text{ and } TTP_2 \text{ is uncensored} \tag{8.2}$$

The test statistic (equivalent to a sign test statistic) is

$$K = \frac{\left(\sum_i r_i \right)^2}{\sum_i r_i^2},$$

has a χ^2 distribution with 1 degree of freedom. For a type I error of 0.05, a power of 80 %, and a 50 % expected correlation between the two consecutive TTP (adjusted for treatment effect), the sample size will be strongly reduced by a factor 4 as compared to the number of patients needed to carry out a randomized comparative trial with the same power.

Case Control Studies

Tsimberidou and colleagues reported their experience from the MD-Anderson phase I unit where outcomes of patients with molecular alteration treated with matched therapy (cases) were compared with those of patients seen during the same period of time, but for whom no matched targeted therapy was available or for whom molecular profile could not be obtained (controls) (Tsimberidou et al. 2014). Multivariate analysis was then carried out to adjust for potential confounders. The results showed an improvement in PFS from 2.2 months to 3.7 months when treated with matched therapy. As in any nonrandomized case control studies, the possibility of matching cases and controls is crucial. In addition to the treatment effect, numerous baseline characteristics as well as follow-up factors may bias the outcome. Multivariate analysis is inherently limited by the collected data, the current knowledge on the prognostic factors, and the patients' allocations.

8.4.3.2 Modular Designs

To control for the heterogeneity in tumor type, the study can be designed as parallel randomized phase II trials. In each of the main histology or for each of the pathways depending on the source of variability we wish to control for, a small-sized phase II is implemented. In each group, decision rules are set up, allowing for interim analysis. This is a flexible approach that may lead to stop early a group (treatment or histology) where the effect is not promising. If all groups are completed, the final analysis will have the planned power to answer the question of the overall benefit of the strategy of sorting patients based on the molecular profile. In addition, evidences of activity per subgroup are collected.

MOST

The MOST trial (NCT02029001) is a good example of this approach in a phase II setting. For each of the investigated treatment, a randomized discontinuation design has been initiated (Ratain et al. 2006). All patients are treated for a period of 16 weeks with the investigational treatment matching the molecular alteration. Patients stable at 16 weeks are randomized between continuing the targeted treatment and switching for treatment at investigator's choice. Accrual in some groups may be longer to complete depending on the prevalence of the alteration in the population. Results of the SHIVA feasibility study (Le Tourneau et al. 2014) reveals that the PI3K/AKT/mTOR pathway was commonly activated in the accrued population, while less than 10 % of the patients had alterations in the MAP kinase pathway. Furthermore, to make the best of the flexibility of such a design, it is necessary that the outcomes data are collected in due time, which is challenging in multi-institution trials. Finally, only massive effects can be detected in each of the subgroups due to the limited sample sizes.

LUNG-MAP

The Lung Cancer Master Protocol (Lung-MAP, NCT02154490) is a multi-arm, biomarker-driven ongoing clinical trial for patients with advanced squamous cell lung cancer sponsored by the South West Oncology Group. Contrary to MOST, this is a phase II/III clinical trial in a unique tumor type. A total of 10,000 patients are planned to be accrued in more than 400 sites in the United States. As described in the clinicaltrials.gov website, "this screening and multi-sub-study randomized phase II/III trial will establish a method for genomic screening of similar large cancer populations followed by assigning and accruing simultaneously to a multi-sub-study "Master Protocol." The type of cancer trait will determine to which sub-study, within this protocol, a participant will be assigned to compare new targeted cancer therapy or combinations to standard of care therapy with the ultimate goal of being able to approve new targeted therapies in this setting. In addition, the protocol includes a "nonmatch" sub-study which will include all screened patients not eligible for any of the biomarker-driven sub-studies. This sub-study will compare a nonmatch therapy to standard of care also with the goal of approval." Spanning from phase II to phase III in each of the five sub-studies will be based on preplanned tests and interim analyses. So each sub-study will function autonomously, will open and close independently, and is independently powered for overall survival (OS) with an interim analysis for progression-free survival (PFS) to determine whether to proceed from phase II into phase III. The statistical theory behind this type of trial is then well established with a strong control of the error rates; controls are well defined and common to all patients within a sub-study, which should allow for drug approval if one or several arms turn out to be more effective than the standard control. This is somehow in contrast with the adaptive designs presented in the next subsection 8.4.3.3.

ACSE Program

An alternative design is to run parallel single-arm phase II trials. This approach was selected to investigate crizotinib and vemurafenib in various tumor types with either *ALK* translocation or V600E *BRAF* mutation in the ACSE program (NCT NCT02034981). For each tumor type, the response rate will be provided. This rate may be difficult to interpret in absence of control arm, especially for rare tumors or in tumors where the prevalence of alteration is low. Pooled analysis can be done to explore toxicity of the agent under study.

8.4.3.3 Adaptive Designs

Previous designs assumed that the algorithm to predict the response to the treatment was known upfront and intangible (at least it should be). This is often unrealistic. For several treatments, no predictive markers have been identified, or a multitude of targets have been characterized as with dasatinib but none being key drivers of the activity. Conversely, predictive factors of response to treatment that have been validated currently consist in single molecular alteration; absence or presence of the alteration is often a necessary but not sufficient condition to obtain individual benefit. Examples include absence of mutation on *KRAS*, *ALK* translocation, etc. Even in these success stories, there is room for improvement in the prediction of response. Therefore, a stimulating idea is to modify the algorithm during the course of the trial based on the data collected so far. Famous examples include the BATTLE (Kim et al. 2011), I-SPY 2 (Barker et al. 2009), or FOCUS 4 trials.

Battle Trial

The objective was to investigate four agents together with 11 molecular alterations (targets) in patients with advanced non-small cell lung cancers that expressed at least one of the targets. The main endpoint was response at eight weeks. The design combined adaptive randomization and Bayesian inference. The hypothesis at the treatment initiation was that any targets had an equal probability to be a predictive factor of response to any of the four agents. Therefore, the first patients entering the trial were randomized between the different treatment arms with a 1/4 probability. During the course of the trial, the data were analyzed before each new inclusion, and the probability of response was calculated for each treatment in presence of each target. The newly accrued patients were then randomized between the various arms in a non-balanced way. The probability to be allocated to a given arm depended on both his (her) molecular alteration and the response probability calculated based on all previous observations. For instance, suppose that at a given time the trial, in presence of an alteration, the estimated probability of activity of erlotinib, vandetanib, erlotinib plus bexarotene, and sorafenib is 10, 20, 25, and 45 %, respectively. A patient with this molecular alteration would be more likely to receive sorafenib. Update in the probabilities of toxicity is done using a Bayesian framework. This concept is appealing but has some strong pitfall. The main one is that the probabilities of toxicity are estimated using few data. As there are 4^{11} possibilities of matching and as many estimates, the risk of error is very high. Therefore, the design is strongly driven by prior information and model calibration. No statistical test procedure can be implemented, and the error estimate has not the same interpretation as in a non-Bayesian framework. Second, the logistic process to get the data in due time is challenging and may lead to severe biases if some outcomes are reported more rapidly than others. Last, the final level of evidence we get varies strongly from treatment to treatment and among targets. Typically, targets with lower prevalences or treatment that appeared less active in the first patients are explored in very few patients; any conclusions are associated with large credibility intervals.

I-SPY 2

The I-SPY 2 study investigated a prognostic algorithm of pathological complete response in stage 3 breast cancer patients. Patients could be randomized between standard neoadjuvant chemotherapy and the same treatment combined with a molecularly targeted agent based on molecular alterations identified on tumor biopsy. The primary endpoint was the pathological complete response rate. Estimates of the probability of pathological response were reassessed in the various treatment arms at several time points; based on these estimates, the protocol allowed opening new treatment arms during the trial or to early close presumably non-efficient treatment arms and to expand promising arms. A Bayesian framework was used to compute the success probability of each arm. This design is close to the approach used in the MOST trial except that adaptation in the investigated arms and in the sample sizes is incorporated.

FOCUS 4

The FOCUS 4 is a phase II/III trial in metastatic colorectal patients (Kaplan et al. 2013). Patients are allocated to one of five maintenance treatment groups depending on the molecular alterations identified. Twenty-four hundred patients will be included with the aim of randomizing 1536 patients. In each treatment arm, patients are randomized against placebo with a 2:1 ratio. An adaptive design is used so that promising treatment arms can switch from a phase II to a phase III and ineffective arms may be dropped prematurely. A substantial advantage of this trial is its ability to include any colorectal cancer patient as molecular stratification covers all molecular subgroups. Adaptation is more conventional as it is essentially a stop and go process embedded in the trial, even if it belongs to the "less well-understood" group of adaptive designs as categorized by the EMA. The very large sample size will provide high levels of evidence compared to previous adaptive designs that were mainly exploratory.

8.5   Conclusions and Challenges

More than 800 MTAs are under development today (America's Biopharmaceutical Research 2014). Many subgroups represent less than 15 % of the cancer patients with a tumor type. Several randomized trials have been set up to investigate which of tumor biology or tumor location and histology is the most important to select treatment in patients with cancer refractory to the standard of care. Interpretation of the results of such trials is complicated by the complexity of the algorithm, but only randomized trials can disentangle the consequence of prognostic factors in these highly selected patients from the intervention effect and enable to control for confounding factors to allow reliable conclusions (Buyse and Michiels 2013). Heterogeneity in the population will be balanced between the two treatment arms and thus should not induce spurious association, but heterogeneity in the treatment effect may dilute the benefit of the intervention. Standardization of the process to identify druggable molecular alterations and the matching MTA, as well as the blinding of the results are key elements in such trials. The same principles as those applied for the development of diagnostic tools should be implemented (Rennie 2003).

There is a need for more sensible endpoints to evaluate such complex interventions. PFS is mildly sensitive to treatment variations, and interaction tests to identify differential effects according to the matching between treatment and target are not powerful with 200 patients. Pharmacodynamic endpoints such as functional imaging or biomarkers are promising to detect early treatment failure but none have yet been validated. Overall, cancer biology is at the heart of this type of histologic-agnostic trial. Current knowledge of tumor biology does not enable us to systematically predict the final outcome as shown by the disappointing efficacy obtained with vemurafenib in *BRAF*-mutated colon cancer (Prahallad et al. 2012) or those obtained with crizotinib in neuroblastoma with *ALK* translocation (Mossé et al. 2013). Taking into account the presence or the absence of several molecular alterations might improve the accuracy of the treatment algorithms using systems biology approaches. However, any treatment algorithm should be clearly defined and rigorously evaluated in randomized trials. In addition, the tumor environment is likely an important factor of success of a therapeutic approach, as illustrated with the recent approval of immunotherapeutics. Nevertheless, the question of what is the strongest predictor of the treatment effect and whether matched MTA to molecular profile compared to conventional chemotherapy is more effective for cancer patients is crucial for the scientific community as well as for the patients.

References

An MW, Mandrekar SJ, Sargent DJ (2013) Application of tumor measurement-based metrics in the real world. J Clin Oncol 31(34):4374

André F, Bachelot T, Commo F et al (2014) Comparative genomic hybridisation array and dna sequencing to direct treatment of metastatic breast cancer: a multicentre, prospective trial (safir01/unicancer). Lancet Oncol 15(3):267–274

Bang YJ, Van Cutsem E, Feyereislova A et al (2010) Trastuzumab in combination with chemotherapy *versus* chemotherapy alone for treatment of *HER2*-positive advanced gastric or gastro-oesophageal junction cancer (ToGA): a phase 3, open-label, randomised controlled trial. Lancet 376(9742):687–697

Barker AD, Sigman CC, Kelloff GJ et al (2009) I-spy 2: an adaptive breast cancer trial design in the setting of neoadjuvant chemotherapy. Clin Pharmacol Ther 86(1):97–100

Boutron I, Estellat C, Guittet L et al (2006) Methods of blinding in reports of randomized controlled trials assessing pharmacologic treatments: a systematic review. PLoS Med 3(10):e425

Buyse M, Michiels S (2013) Omics-based clinical trial designs. Curr Opin Oncol 25(3):289–295

Buyse M, Quinaux E, Hendlisz A et al (2011) Progression-free survival ratio as end point for phase II trials in advanced solid tumors. J Clin Oncol 29(15):e451–e452, author reply e453

Eisenhauer EA, Therasse P, Bogaerts J et al (2009) New response evaluation criteria in solid tumors: revised RECIST guideline (version 1.1). Eur J Cancer 45(2):228–247

Hollebecque A, Massard C, Soria JC (2014) Implementing precision medicine initiatives in the clinic: a new paradigm in drug development. Curr Opin Oncol 26(3):340–346

Horstmann E, McCabe MS, Grochow L et al (2002) Risks and benefits of phase 1 oncology trials, 1991 through 2002. N Engl J Med 352(9):895–904

Jung SH (1999) Rank tests for matched survival data. Lifetime Data Anal 5(1):67–79

Kaplan R, Maughan T, Crook A et al (2013) Evaluating many treatments and biomarkers in oncology: a new design. J Clin Oncol 31(36):4562–4568

Kim ES, Herbst RS, Wistuba II et al (2011) The battle trial: personalizing therapy for lung cancer. Cancer Discov 1(1):44–53

Le Tourneau C, Diéras V, Tresca P et al (2010) Current challenges for the early clinical development of anticancer drugs in the era of molecularly targeted agents. Target Oncol 5(1):65–72. doi:10.1007/s11523-010-0137-6

Le Tourneau C, Servois V, Diéras V (2012) Tumor growth kinetics assessment: added value to RECIST in cancer patients treated with molecularly targeted agents. Br J Cancer 106(5):854–857

Le Tourneau C, Paoletti X, Servant N et al (2014) Randomised proof-of-concept phase II trial comparing targeted therapy based on tumor molecular profiling vs conventional therapy in patients with refractory cancer: results of the feasibility part of the shiva trial. Br J Cancer 111(1):17–24

Litière S, de Vries EGE, Seymour L et al (2014) The components of progression as explanatory variables for overall survival in the Response Evaluation Criteria in Solid Tumors 1.1 database. Eur J Cancer 50(10):1847–1853

McShane LM, Cavenagh MM, Lively TG et al (2013) Criteria for the use of omics-based predictors in clinical trials. Nature 502(7471):317–320

Mick R, Crowley JJ, Carroll RJ (2000) Phase II clinical trial design for noncytotoxic anticancer agents for which time to disease progression is the primary endpoint. Control Clin Trials 21(4):343–359

Mossé YP, Lim MS, Voss SD et al (2013) Safety and activity of crizotinib for paediatric patients with refractory solid tumors or anaplastic large-cell lymphoma: a Children's Oncology Group phase 1 consortium study. Lancet Oncol 14(6):472–480

Olmos D, A'hern RP, Marsoni S et al (2012) Patient selection for oncology phase I trials: a multi-institutional study of prognostic factors. J Clin Oncol 30(9):996–1004

Paoletti X, Mathoulin-Pèlissier S, Michiels S (2011) Facteurs pronostiques et facteurs prèdictifs. In: Mathoulin-Pèlissier S, Kramar A (eds) Méthodes biostatistiques appliquées à la recherche clinique en cancérologie. John Libbey Eurotext, Paris, France. p 382

Prahallad A, Sun C, Huang S et al (2012) Unresponsiveness of colon cancer to BRAF(V600E) inhibition through feedback activation of EGFR. Nature 483(7387):100–103

Presented by America's Biopharmaceutical Research. Medicines in Development – Cancer. 2014. http://catalyst.phrma.org/medicines-in-development-for-cancer-2014

Ratain MJ, Eisen T, Stadler WM et al (2006) Phase II placebo-controlled randomized discontinuation trial of sorafenib in patients with metastatic renal cell carcinoma. J Clin Oncol 24(16):2505–2512

Rennie D (2003) Improving reports of studies of diagnostic tests: the STARD initiative. JAMA 289(1):89–90

Ribba B, Holford NH, Magni P et al (2014) A review of mixed-effects models of tumor growth and effects of anticancer drug treatment used in population analysis. CPT Pharmacometrics Syst Pharmacol 3:e113

Rodon J, Soria JC, Berger R et al (2015) Challenges in initiating and conducting personalized cancer therapy trials: perspectives from WINTHER, a Worldwide Innovative Network (WIN) Consortium trial. Ann Oncol. Apr 23 [Epub ahead of print]

Sargent DJ, Conley BA, Allegra C et al (2005) Clinical trial designs for predictive marker validation in cancer treatment trials. J Clin Oncol 23(9):2020–2027

Tournigand C, André T, Achille E et al (2004) FOLFIRI followed by FOLFOX6 or the reverse sequence in advanced colorectal cancer: a randomized GERCOR study. J Clin Oncol 22(2):229–237

Tsimberidou AM, Wen S, Hong DS et al (2014) Personalized medicine for patients with advanced cancer in the phase I program at MD Anderson: validation and landmark analyses. Clin Cancer Res 20(18):4827–4836

Von Hoff DD, Stephenson JJ, Rosen P et al (2010) Pilot study using molecular profiling of patients' tumors to find potential targets and select treatments for their refractory cancers. J Clin Oncol 28(33):4877–4883

Zalcberg JR, Verweij J, Casali PG et al (2005) Outcome of patients with advanced gastro-intestinal stromal tumors crossing over to a daily imatinib dose of 800 mg after progression on 400 mg. Eur J Cancer 41(12):1751–1757

Chapter 9
Challenges for the Clinical Implementation of Precision Medicine Trials

Maud Kamal

9.1   Introduction

The advent of NGS led in the last few years to a massive increase in cancer molecular profiling and enabled the cataloguing of cancer genomes. The Cancer Genome Atlas and the International Cancer Genomics Consortium have identified recurrent point mutations, translocations, and potentially new therapeutic targets in more than 20 and 50 cancer subtypes, respectively (Hudson et al. 2010). These pioneer projects paved the way for academic cancer centers and companies to translate molecular data to clinical practice. The coevolution of innovative precision medicine (PM) trial designs and sequencing technologies will hopefully provide the data for linking tumor genomics to therapeutic effectiveness. Meanwhile, several challenges need to be overcome to ensure the successful implementation of PM in routine practice.

The first step is the validation of the clinical utility of this approach via well PM designed clinical trials. The setup and conduct of PM trials are associated with numerous challenges including study designs and biomarkers validation, tissue sampling and tumor heterogeneity, standardization of molecular screening techniques, and bioinformatics in the era of continuous technological progress in addition to financial, regulatory, and ethical aspects (Fig. 9.1).

The main objective of PM designs is to identify molecular biomarkers that predict a clinical response (clinical validity) for MTA and to ultimately improve outcomes (clinical utility). PM trials might involve several tumor types, several molecular alterations, and MTAs, which represent a new challenge for biostatisticians. Several designs are today used for this purpose as detailed in chapter 8. Randomized prospective trials are important for patients' follow-up, and data collection, otherwise PFS, is very difficult to interpret with respect to evaluating the effect of a treatment because the rate of PFS of different types of cancer varies

M. Kamal, PhD
Department of Medical Oncology, Institut Curie, Saint-Cloud, Paris, France
e-mail: maud.kamal@curie.fr

© Springer International Publishing Switzerland 2015
C. Le Tourneau, M. Kamal (eds.), *Pan-cancer Integrative Molecular Portrait Towards a New Paradigm in Precision Medicine*,
DOI 10.1007/978-3-319-22189-2_9

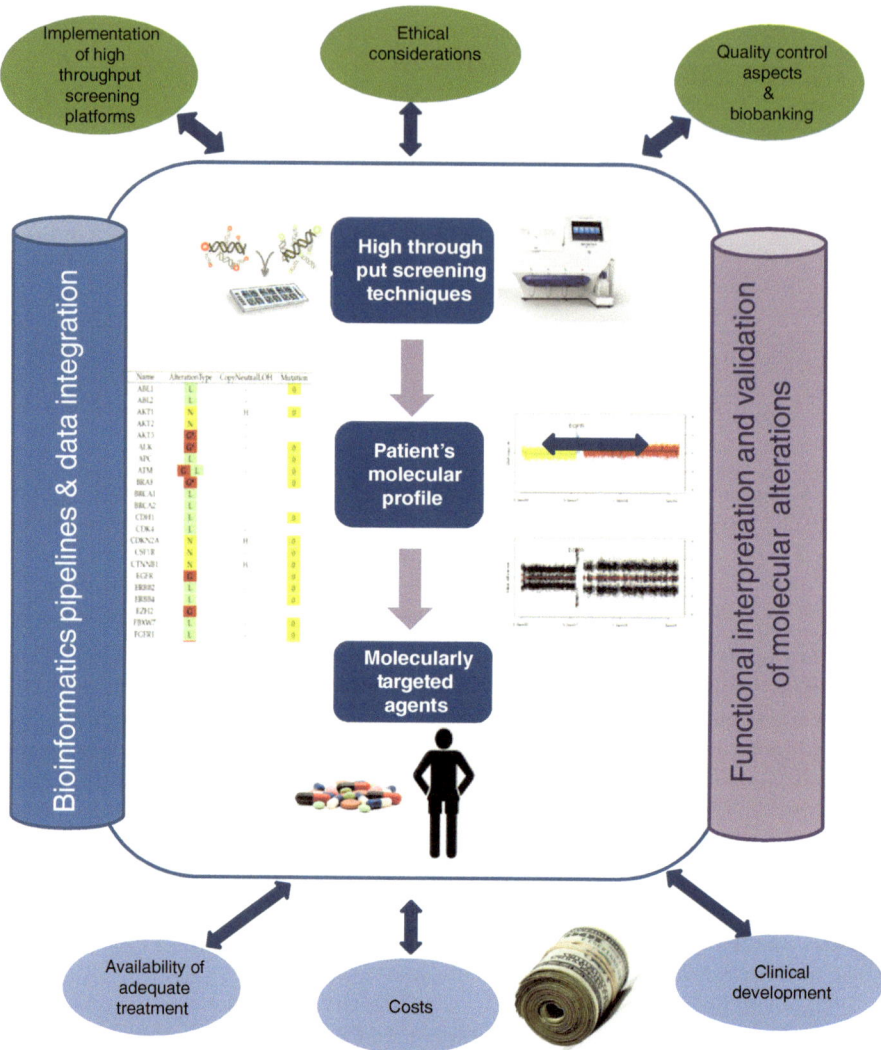

Fig. 9.1 Main challenges associated with precision medicine trials

substantially (Le Tourneau et al. 2014). An ideal design would determine a sample size in order to evaluate treatment effects with enough statistical power in any subgroup of patients with a specific tumor type harboring a specific molecular alteration and treated with a specific treatment. This setup would require thousands of patients and would therefore not be feasible in practice. New trial designs enriched for selected patients to receive a specific treatment, such as randomized discontinuation trials or adaptive randomization, are used today and allow controlling heterogeneity (refer to Chap. 8 for PM trial designs).

PM trials implicate numerous imperative stakeholders, including physicians, radiologists, pathologists, biostatisticians, high-throughput screening platforms managers, bioinformaticians, and biologists. The interactions of these different stakeholders need to be synchronized in order to be able to deliver the appropriate molecular information for patients' treatment.

9.2   Setup of a Precision Medicine Trial: SHIVA Trial Implementation at Institut Curie

The setup and implementation of the SHIVA trial at Institut Curie end of 2012 may provide a realistic example of the challenges behind the setup of this new generation of clinical trials.

The SHIVA trial is the first randomized PM trial worldwide. SHIVA is a multicenter open-label randomized phase II trial involving patients with refractory cancer. In order to randomize and to treat 200 patients, up to 1000 patients were planned to be screened as explained below (Le Tourneau et al. 2014).

Patients meeting selection criteria sign first a consent form in order to perform a biopsy/resection of one metastasis and to establish a molecular profile of their tumor. If no molecular alteration for which an approved matched MTA exists according to a pre-specified treatment algorithm in the frame of the SHIVA trial is identified, patients are not eligible for the randomization and enter into a prospective observational cohort. If one or several molecular alterations are identified, the patient is given a second consent form to sign and has to meet the randomization criteria for randomization.

The setup of SHIVA trial at the French national level required a continuous contact with the clinical research operations, molecular and bioinformatics platforms, biostatisticians and researchers, as well as certified biologists. Several steps following patients' consent necessitated the standardization of the different procedures:

9.2.1   Sample Collection

Standard operating procedures for tissue sampling and biobanking are mandatory for PM trials. In the frame of the SHIVA trial, three tumor samples were required for each patient. One biopsy was fixed and paraffin embedded for diagnostic confirmation as well as estrogen (ER), progesterone (PR), and androgen (AR) receptor expression analyses by IHC. The other biopsies were fresh frozen. One of them was used for DNA extraction using the kit Qiagen® after the evaluation of tumor cell content on a frozen section performed before extraction to allow microdissection of the sample to increase tumor cellularity (refer to Chap. 2 for pathology). Samples containing >30 % of tumor cells were considered suitable for DNA extractions and genomic analyses. This step was performed in all participating centers using a unique protocol. DNA quantity and quality were also assessed before transfer to the molecular platforms. The remaining frozen biopsies were used in case of insufficient DNA amount/quality for molecular analyses or otherwise stored for further studies.

9.2.2   Molecular Analyses

The use of high-throughput screening techniques in PM trial is not a trivial question since it includes a constant and complex interaction between different stakeholders and implicates a synchronized effort from tumor biopsy to result delivery. Several steps need to be standardized to ensure homogeneous procedures for all the patients within the trial and consequently guarantee a potential reproducibility of the results. This quite logical strategy is difficult to actually implement in the absence of clear guidelines for molecular analysis. The molecular profile of each patient enrolled in the SHIVA trial was performed using Ion Torrent/PGM (Life Technologies®) for mutation detection, CytoScan HD (Affymetrix®) for gene copy number alterations, and immunohistochemistry (IHC) for protein expression assessments and amplifications/deletion validation.

Molecular analyses were performed on three different platforms throughout France: Institut Curie, Paris, Centre Léon-Bérard, and Centre René Gauducheau, Nantes.

The majority of the molecular analyses were centralized at Institut Curie for the other recruiting centers. In order to ensure that all analyses were standardized, five DNA samples were processed at the same time on the different platforms for both mutation and gene copy number alteration analyses. The data were then collected and analyzed, and the reproducibility of the results was mandatory for the prospective analyses. In addition, two versions of the AmpliSeq cancer panel were used in the frame of the trial, and the transition to the second version also required a standardization procedure.

Concerning the hormone receptor expression levels, the technique is a routine procedure and consequently was performed by the different centers. For the validation of amplifications and deletions, the IHC was centralized at Institut Curie to ensure homogeneous results. For example, the genomic loss or a deletion of *PTEN* has been performed using a standard procedure for the SHIVA trial (refer to Chap. 2).

9.2.3   Bioinfomatics and Molecular Report

All NGS and CytoScan HD bioinformatics analyses were centralized at the Institut Curie. These analyses were performed within 48 h. Data were stored in a centralized database, along with the results of IHC performed in the Pathology Department. The bioinformatics' platform provided a name-blinded technical report of the

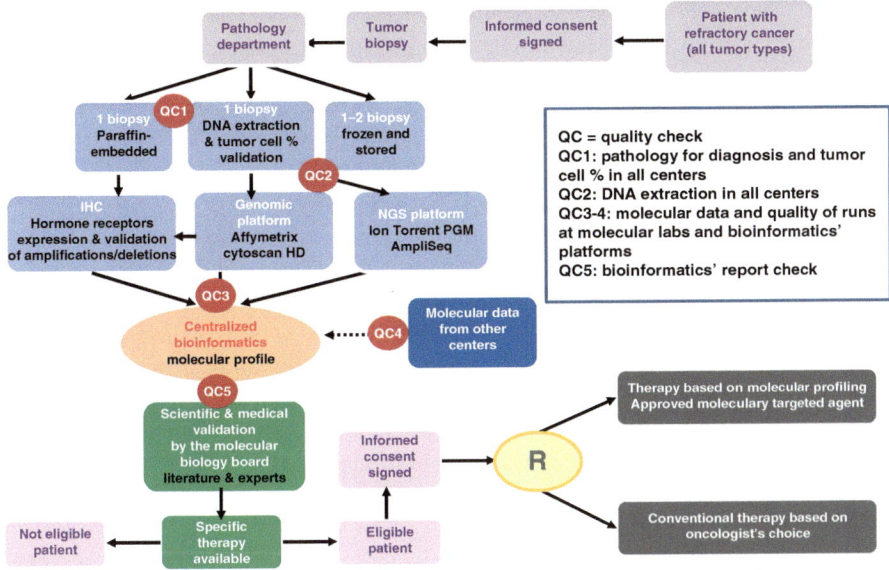

Fig. 9.2 SHIVA trial samples flow and quality checkpoints

different molecular abnormalities identified (mutations, gene copy number alterations, and hormone receptors' expression) to the Molecular Biology Board (MBB) of SHIVA. Automatic and manual controls generate query forms, and any change in the database was tracked. In addition, a seamless information system allowing the integration of the different types of clinical and molecular data was used. This information system ensured data management, data traceability, data analysis, query, and visualization. Being a prospective trial, SHIVA required different checkpoints at different levels from the biopsy to DNA extraction, quality control of the DNA and molecular data, as well as IHC, in order to ensure reproducibility of the results and a real-time follow-up. The molecular data were analyzed only when the checkpoints of the different steps were validated. For example, if the quality of the DNA was bad, the molecular platforms would not process the sample; if the quality of the NGS or CytoScan HD run was not acceptable than the bioinformatics pipeline would not process the data. In addition, only when all the clinical and molecular data were gathered, the bioinformatics' analysis was performed and the report was edited (Fig. 9.2).

One of the main important controls is to ensure the traceability of the patient's samples and data. Thus, any additional quality control which can help in decreasing the sources of technical errors has to be implemented. Among them, a simple quality control can be set for all sequencing runs. The main idea is to be able to detect technical errors within a run, such as wrong patient identification, sample inversion, duplication, or contamination. One simple control which can be applied in practice is to select a list of highly polymorphic SNPs covered by the used sequencing panel. A set of 30 SNPs is usually enough to define a signature which is unique for each patient. This polymorphism signature can be then used to cluster the patient sequenced in the same run and detect any patient duplication. Another systematic control would be to check whether the somatic mutations detected, given one patient, are also detected in the other patients. This control can help detecting contamination or recurrent sequencing artifacts. It is therefore advised, as performed in frame of the SHIVA trial, to create an internal database with recurrent detected mutations which are likely to be false-positive events.

To achieve maximum clinical benefit, molecular results must be reported to clinicians in a clear and easily digestible way, yet with all supporting information necessary to interpret the significance of all molecular alterations that were detected. In this context, a detailed bioinformatics report was edited and provided anonymously to the MBB of the SHIVA trial. The report included few clinical information such as the sex of the patient, the histology type, and previous targeted therapies, necessary to the interpretation of the molecular results. In addition, the report provided a summary of the main alterations on the first pages on the report then a detailed picture of each gene mutational and DNA copy number alterations' status (refer to Fig. 6.16).

9.2.4 Molecular Biology Board: A Treatment Algorithm

A major challenge in optimizing PM trials design is the appropriate use of relevant biomarkers to the MTA(s) in question and in case of several MTAs tested the setup of an appropriate algorithm. It is clear today that functional significance of some molecular alterations may differ across tumor types. Several molecular alterations are also observed in tumors, and few are considered "drivers." The challenge is to be able to decipher the "driver" alterations and among these the alterations of major deleterious impact and those which are the determinants of inherent or acquired resistance in the context where very few alterations are validated in the clinics (refer to chapter 7). This issue is very tricky and complicates the setup of appropriate algorithms in PM trials. Based either on clinical or preclinical evidence, the functional significance of the biomarkers is continuously questioned not necessarily concerning its own function but most probably by the discovery of other alterations that can affect this function. Consequently, the presence of a multidisciplinary MBB is mandatory for all PM trials. The MBB of the SHIVA trial included biologists, physicians, bioinformaticians and the technical platforms' managers, as well as basic and translational researchers. The MBB was in charge of the scientific validation and prioritization of the identified molecular abnormalities. Following the MBB, a final synthetic report was validated and signed by the accredited biologists. Previous therapy was taken into account by the physicians for the treatment recommendation. The whole process was set up in order to have less than 4 weeks elapsed between the biopsy and the day the MBB. The MBB got together on a weekly basis via a teleconference.

MTAs used in the experimental arm of the SHIVA trial were only drugs approved for clinical use in France. Single MTAs were selected following a predefined treatment algorithm (Le Tourneau et al. 2014), except for patients whose tumor harbored a mutation or an amplification of HER-2 who were proposed to be treated with trastuzumab and lapatinib given the overall survival benefit demonstrated in *HER2*-overexpressing metastatic breast cancer patients. The control arm was conventional chemotherapy as per oncologist's choice. SHIVA treatment algorithm has been set up following several meetings with biologist and researchers and took into account the few alterations validated in the clinics and alterations described in the literature in a preclinical setting. In case of several alterations, the prioritization of the molecular alterations was discussed by the MBB based on specific criteria maintained throughout the trial to ensure reproducibility of treatment decision in all patients enrolled. For example, any molecular alteration (mutation, amplification, or deletion) was considered of a higher impact than hormone receptor expression. Only focal amplifications, defined as gene copy number ≥6 for diploid tumors and ≥7 for tetraploid tumors and an amplicon size of ≤10 Mb, are considered in the SHIVA algorithm. The amplifications ranging between 1 and 10 Mb require protein expression confirmed by IHC. Gene losses are defined as one copy for diploid tumors and one or two copies for tetraploid tumors, whereas gene deletions corresponded to zero copy. Losses of tumor suppressor genes such as *PTEN* required a confirmation by IHC of the loss of the protein. However, homozygous deletion did not require any further validation. Non-synonymous and nonrecurrent mutations were considered in the SHIVA algorithm. The MBB decides based on the literature whether or not these mutations are functionally relevant.

In case of two molecular alterations described in the same patient, the MBB discussed the case based on the latest literature review to select the most "relevant" anomaly. In general, alterations with clinical validation such as HER-2 amplification, *BRAF* mutation (V600E), etc., prevail. Well-characterized mutations such as PI3KCA mutations (E542K, E545K/Q, H1047L/R) are also on the top of the list. Resistance biomarkers were not taken onto account except for *EGFR* activation (amplification or activating mutations).

The treatment algorithm was the cornerstone of the SHIVA trial, and the main challenge was to be up to date with the literature without changing the algorithm to ensure that the 200 randomized patients were treated according to the same criteria.

9.3 Tissue Sampling and Tumor Heterogeneity

A major issue for PM in general and PM trial in particular is in what extent the sample used for molecular analysis is representative of the tumor. Several reports actually revealed the huge complexity of the cancer genome as well as a striking heterogeneity in solid tumors. Tumor heterogeneity was confirmed by NGS analyses, which also suggested that it might be the result of a branching evolution of the molecular characteristics of cancer (Meacham and Morrison 2013). Recent comparative studies suggest that molecular alterations found in metastatic samples reflect the patterns of subclones that already exist in the primary tumor. Some of these subclones may also acquire additional mutations that may be correlated to organ-specific metastasis (Gerlinger et al. 2012). Confusing responses to targeted therapies could be explained by tumor heterogeneity (Turner and Reis-Filho 2012), raising again the question of which tumor biopsy is more representative of the cancer and consequently more suitable for molecular analyses.

In colorectal cancer and NSCLC, the high concordance for *KRAS* and *EGFR* mutations, respectively, between the primary tumor and its metastasis (Vakiani et al. 2012; Jakobsen and Sørensen 2012) may explain the significant efficacy results of cetuximab and panitumumab for patients with advanced *KRAS* wild-type colorectal cancer and gefitinib or erlotinib in *EGFR*-mutated lung adenocarcinoma in trials where mutations were screened on archival material rather than on biopsies from a metastasis. However, in advanced refractory cancers, which progressed following multiple lines of treatments, the analysis of archived material to treat the metastatic cancer does not seem to be appropriate.

PM clinical trials tend to include molecular analysis and usually require a biopsy from a metastatic site, although some might use as well archival material. The latest reports clearly show that taking biopsies of metastatic sites are safe and feasible (Le Tourneau et al. 2014); however, this procedure is not implemented in routine patients' care. In addition certain metastatic sites might not always be easily accessible for sampling, while some are not useful for high-throughput screening techniques for technical reasons.

It is clear today that a single biopsy from a single metastatic site does not seem to be representative of the metastatic cancer and multiple biopsies are definitely not acceptable today in terms of patients' safety and multiplication of the molecular analyses costs, especially that there is no evidence that this strategy can improve PM approaches. More importantly, the MTAs on the market today were able to improve patients' outcome as illustrated by *HER2*-targeting agents in *HER2*-overexpressing breast cancer patients in the metastatic and in the adjuvant settings without taking into account tumor heterogeneity. Circulating (ct) DNA analysis is clearly a potential alternative and/or replacement to analyses using costly, harmful, and lengthy tissue biopsies of metastasis, irrespective of cancer type and metastatic site, for multiplexed mutation detection in selecting MTAs based on the patient's tumor genetic content (Lebofsky et al. 2015).

9.4 Ethical Aspects

PM trials usually include analyses of constitutional DNA for appropriate exome or genome sequencing raising several questions concerning how to deal with incidental findings, such as germline mutations associated with risk for other diseases and those that provide risk information relevant to family members (such as mutations in *BRCA1*/BRCA2). Informed consents have therefore to anticipate these complex issues to ensure the complete comprehension of patients. Patients' advocacy groups become today a major player in PM development and implementation.

9.5 Costs and Drugs Availability

The costs of high-throughput technologies exponentially decreased over the last few years, yet the overall cost of PM trials remains high due to clinical trials' logistics, regulatory aspects, and above all drugs' cost. Data storage is also very expensive, and the increase in data generation is a serious challenge for PM implementation in routine clinic. The implementation of high-throughput technologies within the infrastructure of medical centers and hospitals needs to be precisely analyzed for cost-effectiveness. A possibility is to outsource these analyses, and the main challenge would be to ensure high-quality interpretation of the results, an expertise usually available in comprehensive cancer centers and academic research centers. Discussions not only with health authorities but also with pharmaceutical companies will have to be engaged to discuss cost sharing. Pharmaceutical companies may indeed derive benefits from such implementations that allow patients to be guided in specific molecular-based clinical trials.

Access to drugs represents an important issue for PM trials, especially when several drugs are used. Pharmaceutical companies may not be very interesting in providing their drugs in multidrugs trials, especially that PM clinical trials do not directly benefit pharmaceutical companies, since these trials evaluate algorithms and not drugs' efficacy. Although, indirect benefits might be generated by the use of patients' molecular profile to increase the inclusion rate in clinical trials based on specific molecular alterations.

9.6 Rapid Evolution of High-Throughput Screening Techniques and Bioinformatics

NGS has revolutionized the field of genomics for the last 10 years. Sequencing of whole genomes or transcriptomes, large sample sets in short turnaround time, and reasonable cost have had a huge impact on scientific research and clinical genetic testing (refer to Chap. 4). Nevertheless, the actual second generation of sequencers suffers from limitations and biases that need to be fixed in order to get at least one gold standard technology.

Molecular results are returned to patients and are used for treatment decisions and consequently are subject to legal obligations designed to ensure that tests are reproducible and adhere to high standards of sensitivity and specificity. Molecular platforms need therefore to be validated, and even if guidelines are lacking today, major clinical trials use CLIA-certified platforms to ensure reproducibility of their results. In addition, the National Cancer Institute, in collaboration with scientists representing multiple areas of expertise relevant to "omics"-based test development, has developed a checklist of criteria that can be used to determine the readiness of omics-based tests for guiding patient care in clinical trials (McShane et al. 2013).

The rapid evolution of the high-throughput screening techniques within a few months needs to be taken into consideration for PM trials, simply because the technique used initially might not be available anymore.

The quality of molecular analyses depends on several factors, including the tissue quality, the tumor content within a sample, the depth of sequencing, and the effectiveness of the computational pipeline. The depth of sequencing is directly proportional to the sensitivity of detecting mutations in heterogeneous tissue samples and thus can be adjusted for samples with limited tumor content. The computational pipeline needs to ensure a secure storage of large data files as well as access to high-performance computing to enable rapid analysis of data. The accuracy of variant detection is strongly influenced by the quality of the computational pipeline to avoid false-positive variants' detection (Simon and Roychowdhury 2013). Once the bioinformatics analyses are finalized, the interpretation of the results and the functional validity of each alteration still require a "manual" check by experts committee in light of the latest publications (refer to Chap.7). The integration of different types of data including clinical and molecular is also a major challenge before the actual analyses and report of the results in a digest format that is expected to facilitate data interpretation and treatment decision. PM trials therefore require a strong bioinformatics environment capable of warranting the integration and the traceability of data, ensuring the correct processing and analyses of genomic data, and applying well-defined and reproducible procedures for workflow management and decision-making as illustrated by Servant et al. in the context of the SHIVA trial (Servant et al. 2014, refer to Chap. 6). Maintaining an efficient bioinformatics workflow in a clinical context is today challenging because of the frequent updates of the computational solutions either installed on the sequencing machine or provided as stand-alone applications. These frequent updates are mainly due to the rapid evolution of the sequencing and microarray technologies but remain a major issue to ensure the operability of the bioinformatics pipelines and their reproducibility. As a consequence, any update requires each bioinformatics pipeline to be validated to ensure a high specificity and sensitivity. Any change in the data format or in the analysis methods can have critical consequences on the downstream analysis and results. Moreover, many different methods are currently available to analyze NGS data, but no consensus or standard computational tools exist so far.

Current NGS techniques expand from targeted sequencing based on a couple of genes to exome or whole genome sequencing. The latter is today mainly used in cancer research and can be seen as the future of the clinical investigation. However, their use in routine clinical practice is much more difficult, mainly because the average depth of coverage is much lower than for targeted gene sequencing complicating mutation detection. These applications offer new ways to explore Copy numver variants (CNVs) and can thus be used as an alternative to the current microarray technologies. In addition, the current sequencing strategies offer new opportunities to develop gene/transcript expression and epigenomics biomarkers in clinic. Integrative analysis considering together genome, proteome, and epigenome is a major challenge to explore the complexity of the disease and to identify new therapeutic targets.

9.7 Conclusions

PM trials aim to assess the feasibility of molecular profiling of the tumor for patients' treatment but more importantly to show that treatment based on molecular alteration leads to better clinical outcomes. The continuous progress in high-throughput screening technologies and bioinformatics is crucial to elucidate the different mechanisms and networks underlying cancer development and consequently facilitates the selection of targeted drugs and combinations for a more personalized cancer treatment. The future looks promising, yet several challenges including tumor heterogeneity and the emergence of resistance mechanisms as well as the complexity and influence of the epigenome need to be overcome before the actual implementation of precision medicine in routine oncology. The progress of the high-throughput techniques in an amazing speed will hopefully facilitate the study of cancer stem cells, tumor subclones and components of the adjacent tumor microenvironment (TME), and immune mechanisms. Several international projects assessing epigenomic events in human cancers and how genetic mechanisms affect epigenetic effectors are currently ongoing, but it remains to be demonstrated that epigenetic profiling by using deep sequencing can predict drug response (Sandoval and Esteller 2012).

Recent data show an impressive clinical activity of immune-checkpoint pathway inhibitors such as anti-CTLA-4 (ipilimumab) (Hodi et al. 2010) and anti-programmed death 1 (PD-1) and its ligand (PD-L1) (Topalian et al. 2012; Topalian et al. 2014) monoclonal antibodies in a variety of solid tumors, emphasizing the fact that not all actionable/druggable cancer targets are genomic alterations. Combinations of MTAs and novel therapies such as immunotherapy and therapies targeting the TME seem to have a great potential to treat cancer.

To counter tumor heterogeneity, liquid biopsies definitely present a priceless advantage since they can safely allow sequential sampling with the promise of identifying pharmacodynamic biomarkers of efficacy as well as resistance biomarkers.

With the continuous flow of data from these programs and the advanced bioinformatics' and systems biology approaches, the identification of key signaling pathways and predictive biomarkers for treatment response will soon be available. It remains to be demonstrated that a systems biology approach can improve the patients' outcome. Meanwhile, PM trials need to include a fixed algorithm that could be enriched with new information from recent publications without changing treatment decisions to ensure reproducible results.

Cost-effectiveness analyses also need to be performed to assess the feasibility of the actual implementation of PM in medical facilities. Data storage limitations and the rapid evolution of molecular technologies and bioinformatics' development strategies constitute a daily challenge in providing digest synthetic information to clinicians in order to facilitate treatment decisions.

References

Gerlinger M, Rowan AJ, Horswell S et al (2012) Intratumor heterogeneity and branched evolution revealed by multiregion sequencing. N Engl J Med 366(10):883–892

Hodi FS, O'Day SJ, McDermott DF et al (2010) Improved survival with ipilimumab in patients with metastatic melanoma. N Engl J Med 363(8):711–723

Hudson TJ et al (2010) International Cancer Genome Consortium. International network of cancer genome projects. Nature 464(7291):993–998. Erratum in: Nature 465(7300):966

Jakobsen JN, Sørensen JB (2012) Intratumor heterogeneity and chemotherapy-induced changes in *EGFR* status in non-small cell lung cancer. Cancer Chemother Pharmacol 69(2):289–299

Le Tourneau C, Paoletti X, Servant N et al (2014) Randomised proof-of-concept phase II trial comparing targeted therapy based on tumour molecular profiling vs conventional therapy in patients with refractory cancer: results of the feasibility part of the SHIVA trial. Br J Cancer 111(1):17–24

Lebofsky R, Decraene C, Bernard V et al (2015) Circulating tumor DNA as a non-invasive substitute to metastasis biopsy for tumor genotyping and personalized medicine in a prospective trial across all tumor types. Mol Oncol 9(4):783–790. doi:10.1016/j.molonc.2014.12.003

McShane LM, Cavenagh MM, Lively TG et al (2013) Criteria for the use of omics-based predictors in clinical trials. Nature 502(7471):317–320

Meacham CE, Morrison SJ (2013) Tumour heterogeneity and cancer cell plasticity. Nature 501(7467):328–337

Sandoval J, Esteller M (2012) Cancer epigenomics: beyond genomics. Curr Opin Genet Dev 22(1):50–55

Servant N, Roméjon J, Gestraud P, La Rosa P, Lucotte G, Lair S, Bernard V, Zeitouni B, Coffin F, Jules-Clément G, Yvon F, Lermine A, Poullet P, Liva S, Pook S, Popova T, Barette C, Prud'homme F, Dick JG, Kamal M, Le Tourneau C, Barillot E, (2014) Hupé P.Bioinformatics for precision medicine in oncology: principles and application to the SHIVA clinical trial. Front Genet. 30;5:152. doi:10.3389/fgene.2014.00152. eCollection 2014. Review.

Simon R, Roychowdhury S (2013) Implementing personalized cancer genomics in clinical trials. Nat Rev Drug Discov 12(5):358–369

Topalian SL, Hodi FS, Brahmer JR et al (2012) Safety, activity, and immune correlates of anti-PD-1 antibody in cancer. N Engl J Med 366(26):2443–2454

Topalian SL, Sznol M, McDermott DF et al (2014) Survival, durable tumor remission, and long-term safety in patients with advanced melanoma receiving nivolumab. J Clin Oncol 32(10):1020–1030

Turner NC, Reis-Filho JS (2012) Genetic heterogeneity and cancer drug resistance. Lancet Oncol 13(4):e178–e185

Vakiani E, Janakiraman M, Shen R et al (2012) Comparative genomic analysis of primary *versus* metastatic colorectal carcinomas. J Clin Oncol 30(24):2956–2962